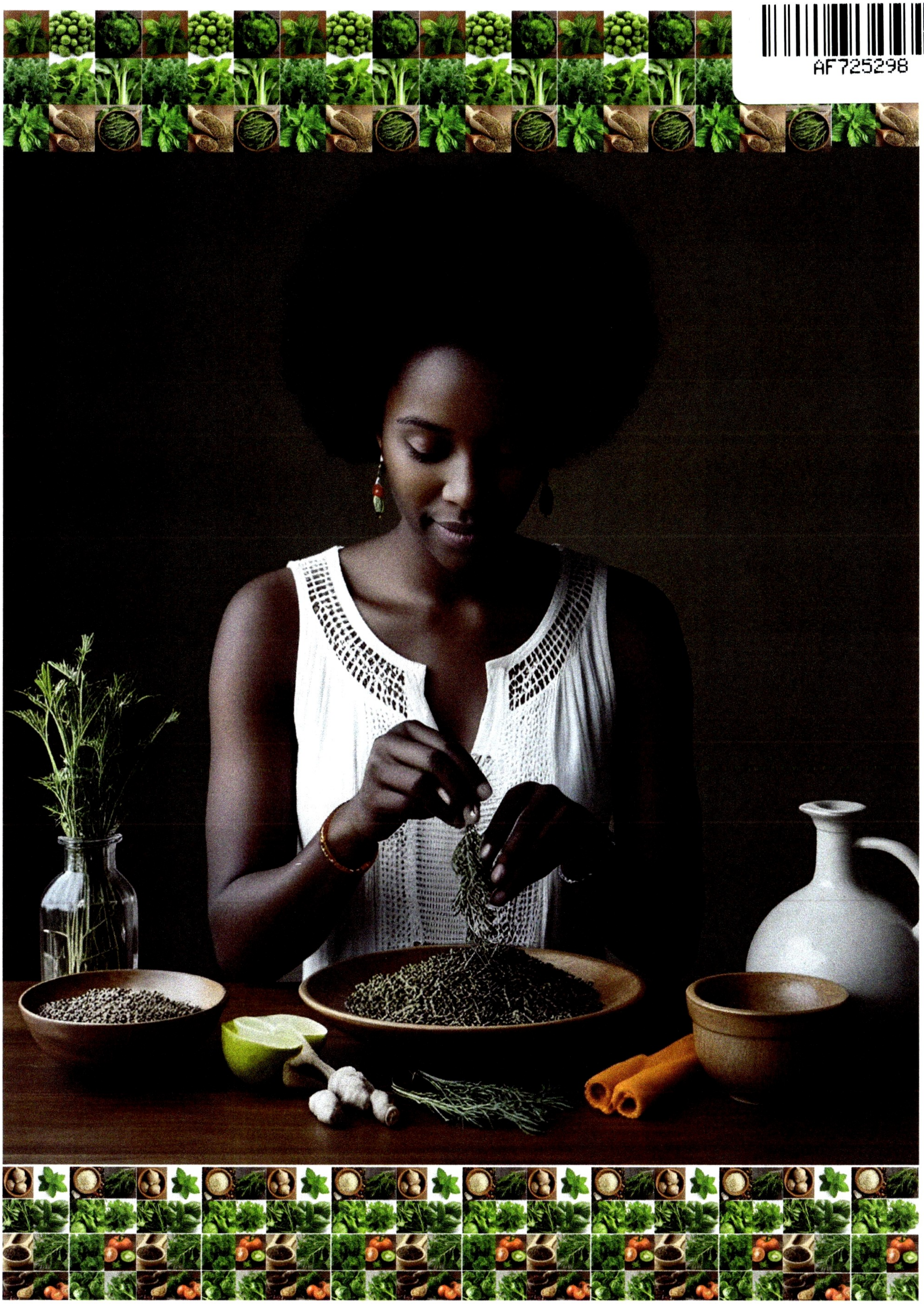

For permission requests, write to the publisher:
Peter-Gaye's Publishing
Email: wordsofpeace30@gmail.com

ISBN: 979-8-3494-7228-2
Printed in: United States
First Edition: 2025

Eternal Life in Plants

Natural remedies in this book offer pure healling

Peter-Gaye's
PUBLISHING

By Donovan Broderick

TABLE OF CONTENTS

Introduction

In a world where pharmaceuticals often take center stage, more and more people are turning to nature in search of safer, gentler paths to healing. Eternal Life in Plants is your guide to the timeless wisdom of plant-based remedies—drawn from the rich herbal traditions of the Caribbean and inspired by natural healing practices from across the globe.

This book explores the incredible power of herbs to support the body, boost immunity, and restore balance—without the harsh side effects of synthetic medications. From calming teas and nourishing infusions to potent plant therapies, Eternal Life in Plants equips you with the knowledge to use nature's medicine with confidence and care.

Whether you're looking to ease digestive discomfort, strengthen your immune defenses, or simply live a more holistic lifestyle, this guide offers practical, accessible remedies to help you on your wellness journey. Step into the world of herbal healing and embrace a natural way to thrive.

Author’s Note

"The herbs and plants mentioned in this book have been widely used in traditional medicine and supported by various studies for their potential health benefits. While many people have experienced positive effects, individual results may vary. This information is provided for educational purposes and should not replace professional medical advice. Consult a healthcare provider before using herbal remedies, especially if you have pre-existing conditions or are taking medication."

Black Sage

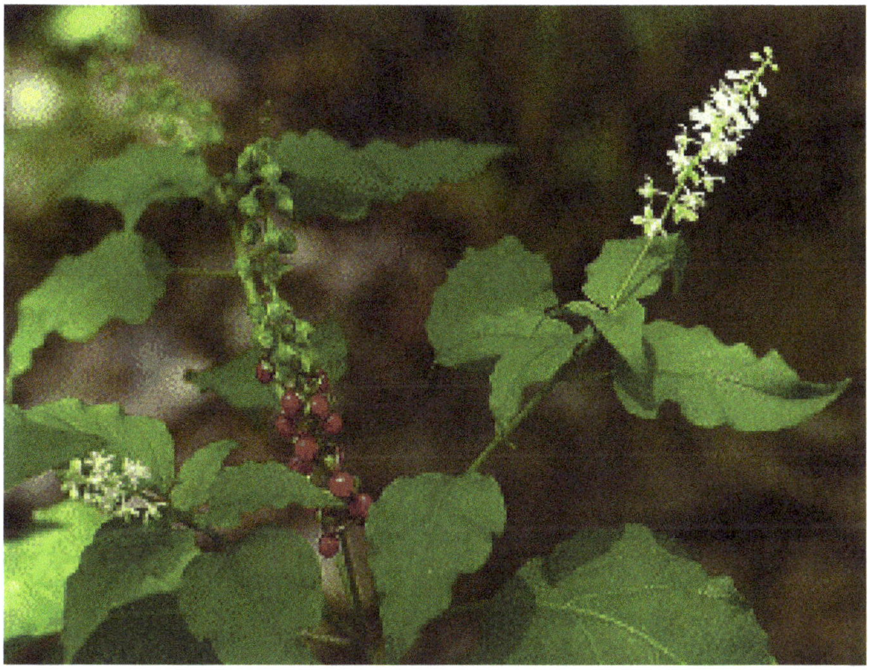

Caribbean herbalists use black sage, also called bloodberry, as a tea for colds and chest tightness or congestion, and it is often combined with the herbs "jack in the bush" and "search mi heart". It is commonly used for menstrual cramps, which might explain one of its names, bloodberry.
It is still used as an astringent for spots and boils, and in Trinidad to treat a range of skin diseases.

In the Brazilian Amazon indigenous people make an infusion from the leaves to treat infections, inflammations, rheumatism and arthritis. It is taken internally or topically.

Its anti-inflammatory properties have been confirmed in the laboratory, and it has been tested as an anti-fungal and larvicidal (anti-mosquito).
The smooth bark is chestnut colored, and the leaves are dark and rough, smelling of citrus.
It thrives in open areas such as fields and pastures, along roads and in open forest. Birds eat the fruits and help spread the seeds in their droppings.
Black sage is not related to the culinary herb we know in Britain as sage (Salvia genus).

To make black sage tea, follow these steps.

Ingredients:

- 1-2 teaspoons of dried black sage leaves (or a few fresh leaves)
- 1 cup of hot water
- Honey or lemon (optional)

Instructions:

1. Boil Water – Bring 1 cup of water to a boil.
2. Add Black Sage – Place the dried or fresh leaves in a cup or teapot.
3. Steep – Pour the hot water over the leaves and let it steep for 10-15 minutes to extract the beneficial compounds.
4. Strain – Remove the leaves by straining the tea.
5. Enhance Flavor – Add honey or lemon if desired.
6. Drink Warm – Sip slowly and enjoy its soothing effects.

Benefits of Black Sage Tea:

- Helps with respiratory health (clears congestion)
- Supports relaxation and sleep
- Aids digestion
- Contains antioxidant and anti-inflammatory properties

Aloe Vera

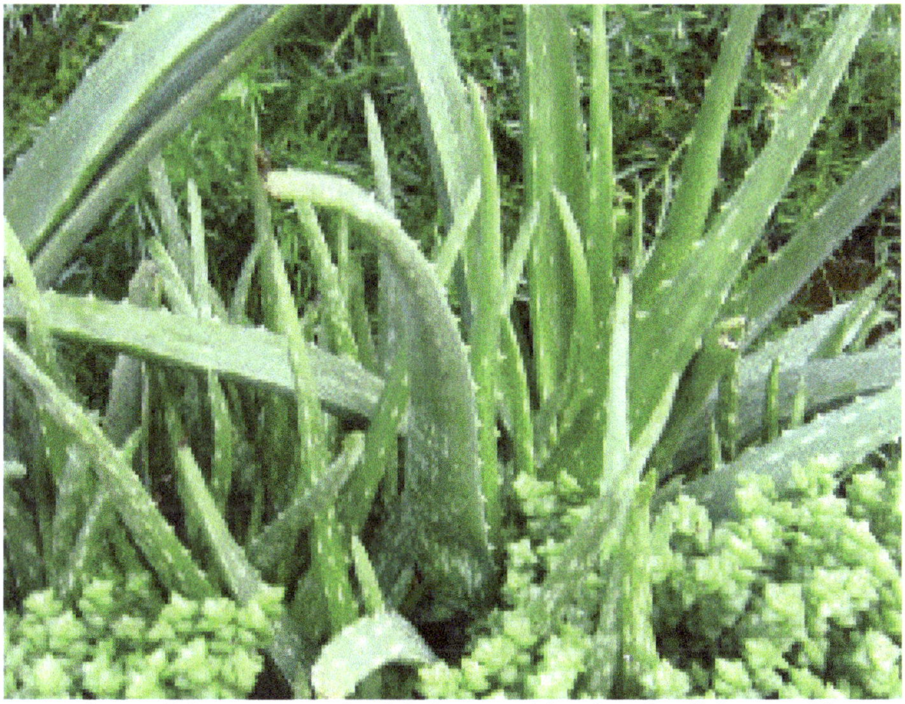

Aloe is extremely well known and widely used in the Caribbean. The cut leaves are steeped in water to extract the slimy pulp and make a drink, as a digestive cleanser and for bilious attacks. It can be very potent, and must be taken with care.

For colds, the leaf is peeled, cut up and steeped in proof rum. The split leaf is applied to wounds, and to the head for headaches.

Aloe is also an additive to hand lotions and skin care products and is used to soothe sunburn, minor burns, wrinkles, insect bites, skin irritations, cuts and scratches. However, it can cause dermatitis in some people.

The plant thrives in warm, dry, sunny habitats. It is thought to have come originally from Africa, but is now found all over the world. It makes a good houseplant if given plenty of sunlight and not over-watered.

Aloe vera can be consumed in several ways, but it's important to prepare it correctly to avoid consuming the latex, which can be harsh on the digestive system. Here's how you can consume aloe vera safely:

1. **Aloe Vera Juice**

- Cut a fresh aloe vera leaf and wash it thoroughly.
- Slice the leaf open and scoop out the clear gel inside.
- Blend the gel with water, coconut water, or fruit juice.
- Strain and drink in moderation (about 1-2 tablespoons per day).

2. **Aloe Vera Smoothie**

- Blend aloe vera gel with fruits like mango, banana, or berries.
- Add honey or lemon juice for extra flavor.
- Drink fresh for a refreshing health boost.

3. **Aloe Vera Tea**

- Add a small amount of aloe vera gel to warm herbal tea.
- Mix well and drink to aid digestion.

4. **Aloe Vera in Salads**

- Cut aloe vera gel into small cubes and mix it into fruit or vegetable salads.

Cerasee

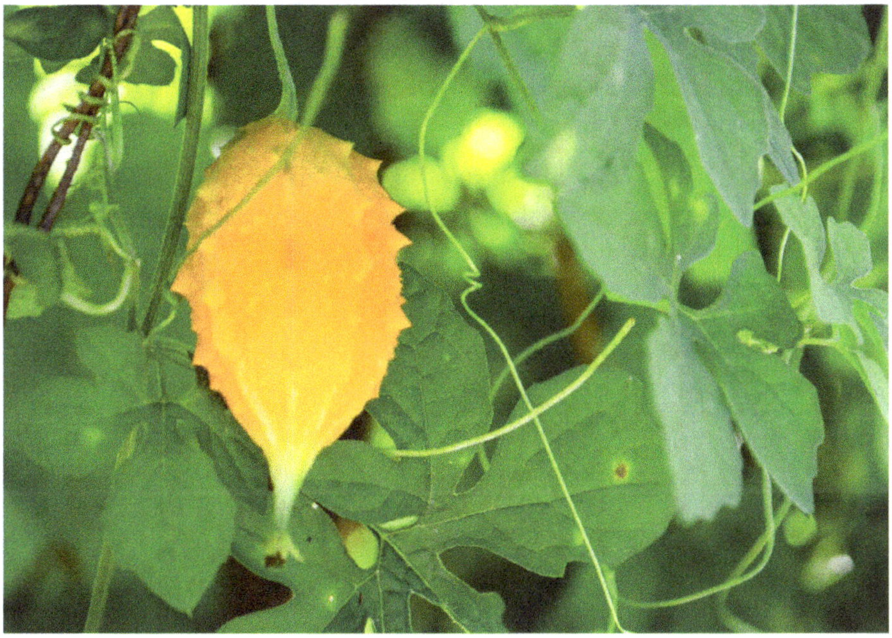

Cerassee (momordica charantia), also known as bitter melon is a very popular herb in Jamaica, feared by many because of its bitterness. It is believed to be a blood cleanser and sugar control agent for diabetes. It is widely accepted that a fair amount of consumption of this tea on a weekly basis will prevent colds, flu, headaches, jaundice, and stomach ache. Cerassee is extremely bitter, and a ghastly tasting but beneficial Jamaican herb.

Cerassee tea may be sweetened with honey or maple syrup. This medicinal herb which is used in Jamaica and many other tropical and sub-tropical countries around the world is still revered by many.

The bush grows wild, unaided by human device. Though it produces pretty bright, yellow flowers and an orange-coloured fruit, it is often viewed as no more than a nuisance, creeping through the garden. Tea brewed from the leaves is popular among rural folk but considered too bitter by most Jamaicans.

Traditional Indian, Chinese and African pharmacopeia, however, for centuries have appreciated the value of this vine-type plant Cerassee (also called Bitter melon, Karela, Balsam pear) has pride of place as a laxative, anthelminthic and an abortifacient. Reports are that even in some of the most modern hospitals in India, Cerassee is dispensed so confident are their doctors about the herb's positive effects on diabetics.

In more recent times, scientists have identified and extracted several active proteins from Cerassee including MAP-30, alpha-momorcharin and beta-momorcharin which have indicated putative value as anti-HIV agents.

The Memorial Sloan Kettering Cancer Center cites that several active substances in bitter melon have been studied in both animals and humans. These experiments show that these substances act in the same way as insulin, by increasing the entry of glucose into cells and promoting its processing and storage in the liver, muscle, and fat. Bitter melon also prevents the conversion of stored nutrients to glucose and the release of this glucose into the blood.

Bitter melon extracts were shown to kill leukemia cells in the laboratory and slow the growth of breast cancer in mice, but it is unknown whether these effects occur in humans. A study in humans showed bitter melon had little effect on the immune system of cervical cancer patients.

Of it's purported benefits, Sloan Kettering also summarizes the following

Prevention of cancer

Laboratory studies show that bitter melon extracts can kill certain cancer cells, but it has not been studied in cancer patients.

Treatment of type 2 diabetes

A few small clinical trials show that bitter melon extracts can lower blood glucose levels, but larger and better-designed clinical trials are needed to fully support this use.

To reduce fever

No scientific evidence supports this use.

Treatment of HIV and AIDS

Preliminary laboratory studies show that bitter melon can slow the ability of HIV to insert its genes into human chromosomes.

Cerasee Tea (Most Common Way)

Ingredients:

- A handful of fresh leaves or vines, or 1–2 tsp dried cerasee
- 1–2 cups water
- Instructions:
- Bring the water to a boil.
- Add cerasee leaves/vines.
- Let it simmer for 5–10 minutes.
- Strain and serve warm or cool.
- Optionally, add a bit of honey or lime to cut the bitterness.

Guinea Hen Weed

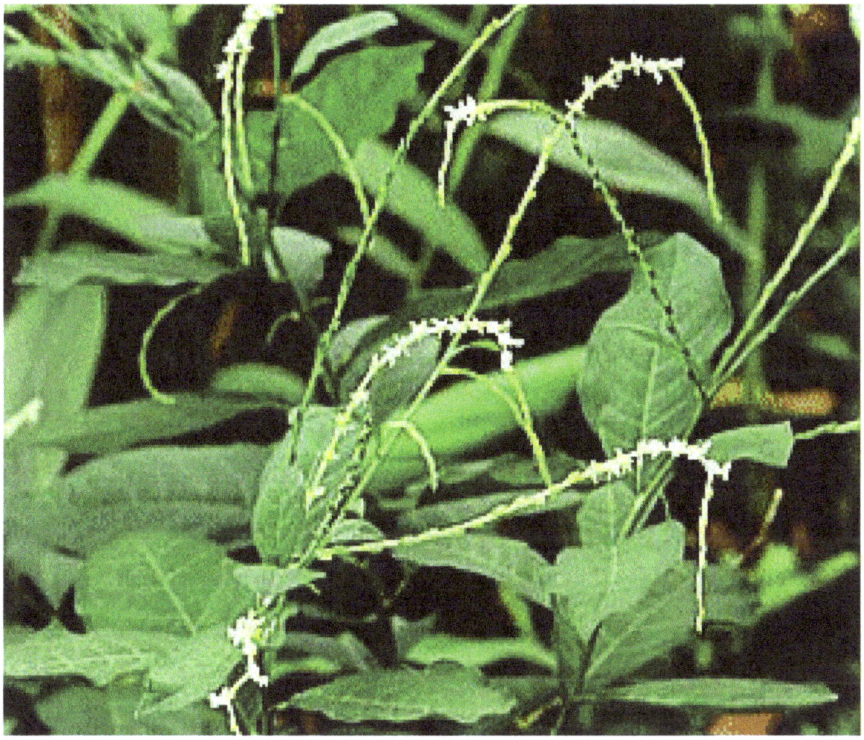

Guinea hen weed is found in the Amazon rainforest and tropical areas of Central and South America, the Caribbean, Africa and some southern states of the US such as Florida. It has a long history as a medicinal plant in the Amazon, where it is known as Anamu. Its main use is for colds and as a pain reliever for headaches, rheumatism and arthritis.

The plant is said to have magical powers and is commonly used in magic rituals. The root is said to be more powerful than the leaves. The strong smelling leaves would be scattered around the room to "to keep away duppies" (unfriendly spirits).
The root is traditionally used in an insecticide preparation, probably because of its strong smell.

Guinea hen weed has been widely studied in the laboratory. Its traditional use for arthritis and rheumatism has been supported by research, which shows it does have anti-inflammatory properties and may stimulate the immune system.
Plant-screening tests have also shown that it contains chemicals active against some types of cancer cells, including forms of leukaemia and breast cancer, although the effect varies. Other studies claim it is active against many strains of bacteria, viruses, fungi and yeast.

Guinea Hen Weed (Petiveria alliacea), also known as Anamu, is a powerful medicinal herb with various health benefits. It is commonly used for its anti-inflammatory, immune-boosting, and pain-relieving properties. Here are some ways to consume it:

1. Guinea Hen Weed Tea (Most Common Method)

Ingredients:

- 1 to 2 teaspoons of dried Guinea Hen Weed leaves, stems, or roots
- 2 cups of water

Instructions:

- Boil the water.
- Add the dried herb and let it simmer for 10–15 minutes.
- Remove from heat, let it cool slightly, then strain.
- Drink 1 cup per day, or as recommended.
- You can add honey or ginger to improve the taste.

2. Guinea Hen Weed Powder (Capsules or Loose Powder)

Instructions:

- Take 1/4 to 1/2 teaspoon of powdered Guinea Hen Weed mixed in warm water, juice, or smoothies.
- If using capsules, follow the dosage on the package (typically one to two capsules per day).

3. Guinea Hen Weed Tincture

Instructions:

- Take 1–2 dropperfuls (around 30–60 drops) of Guinea Hen Weed tincture under the tongue or in a glass of water, 1–2 times daily.

4. Fresh Leaves or Roots (For External Use)

- Crush fresh leaves and apply them directly to the skin for pain relief or as a natural insect repellent.
- Use crushed roots in a poultice for skin infections or inflammation.

Spanish Needles

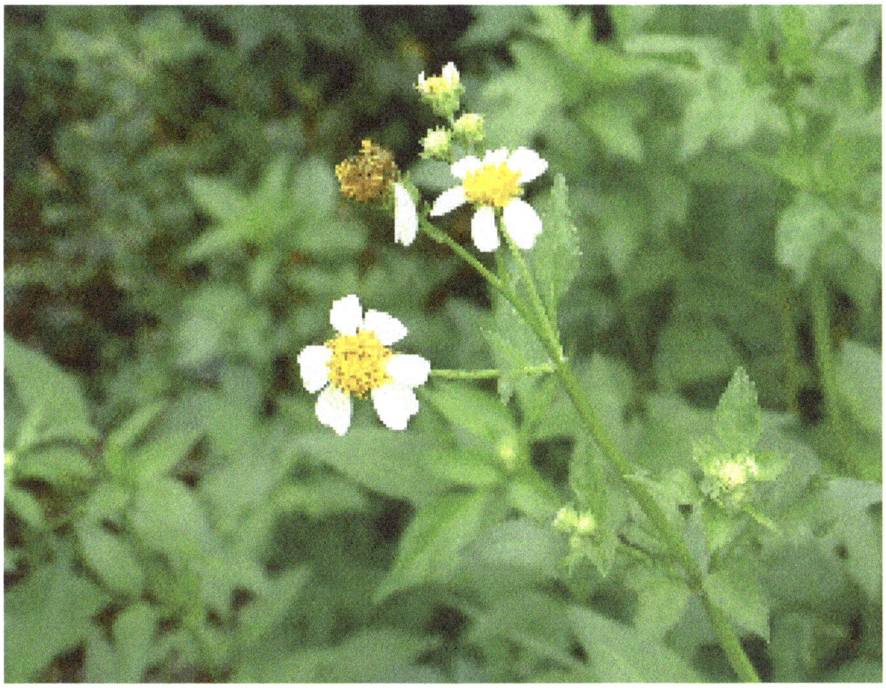

Spanish needles is well-known as a medicinal herb in the Caribbean, as well as in South America and parts of Africa. In Jamaica, they make a tea from the leaves (or the flowers soaked in rum) for colds and toothache. For colic or worms they prepare a mixed infusion of leaves and root.

Spanish needles grow in damp spots, along pasture margins and stream banks. It is native to tropical America, but has spread across all tropical regions and has become one of the world's worst weeds.

Its roots are said to ooze chemicals that hinder other plants growing close to it. Its hooked seeds attach easily to clothing and fur, which helps it spread.
This plant can be confused with its close relative Bidens alba, but the flowers of that species have white ray florets.

In laboratory tests, extracts of this plant have been shown to kill malarial parasites. Interestingly, there are traditional records of its use as an anti-malarial remedy in the Amazon. Lab tests also show antibacterial activity.

Health Benefits of Spanish Needle (Bidens pilosa)

Spanish Needle, also known as Bidens pilosa, is a powerful medicinal plant with numerous health benefits. It is widely used in herbal medicine for its anti-inflammatory, antibacterial, and immune-boosting properties.

1. Boosts the Immune System

- Contains antioxidants and compounds that help strengthen immunity.
- Helps fight infections and promotes faster healing.

2. Anti-Inflammatory Properties

- Reduces inflammation in the body, making it beneficial for conditions like arthritis and joint pain.

3. **Supports Digestive Health**

- Helps relieve stomach issues such as indigestion, ulcers, and bloating.
- Acts as a mild laxative, promoting regular bowel movements.

4. **Controls Blood Sugar Levels**

- Research suggests it may help lower blood sugar levels, making it beneficial for people with diabetes.
- Drinking Spanish Needle tea regularly can aid in blood sugar management.

5. **Wound Healing & Skin Care**

- The leaves and flowers have antibacterial properties that help heal wounds, cuts, and sores.
- Can be applied as a poultice or wash to treat skin infections.

How to Use Spanish Needle

- Tea: Steep fresh or dried leaves in hot water for 10-15 minutes and drink.
- Poultice: Crush fresh leaves and apply to wounds, rashes, or inflamed areas.
- Juice: Blend fresh leaves with water and consume in small amounts.

Moringa

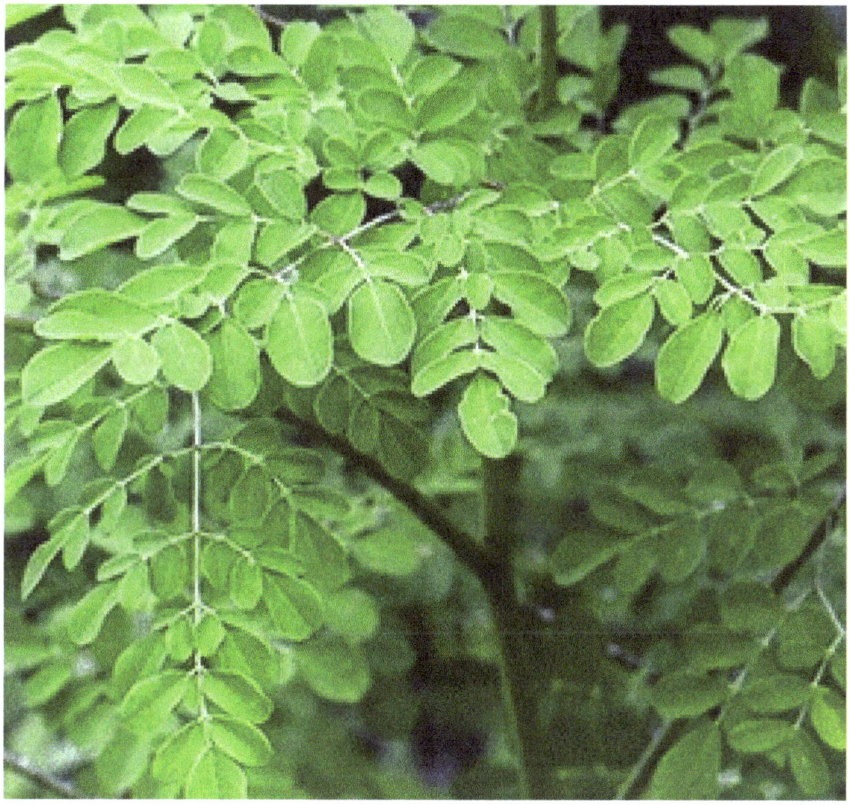

Moringa oleifera is a native plant to northern India. It is popularly called "Moringa" and is known in Jamaica as the drumstick tree, horseradish tree, benzoil tree and the "miracle tree" in some countries. It is also found in other tropical and sub-tropical places such as Asia, Africa, the Caribbean, Central and South America. The leaves, flowers, seeds, and roots of this plant has been used in traditional medicine for centuries.

The plant contains many important vitamins and minerals. The leaves have 7 times the amount of vitamin C as oranges and 15 times more potassium than bananas. It also has calcium, protein, iron, and amino acids that aids the body to heal and build muscle. It is packed with antioxidants that can protect cells from damage and may boost your immune system. There's some evidence that some of these antioxidants can also lower blood pressure and reduce fat in the blood and body.

Traditional Uses

It has been traditionally used for conditions such as:

- Diabetes
- Long-lasting inflammation
- Bacterial, viral, and fungal infections
- Joint pain
- Heart health
- Cancer

Research

1. exactly how the extracts from this plant affect people, but early studies however, shows it may help with the following: Rheumatoid arthritis: Moringa leaf extract may lower fluid swelling, redness, and pain.
2. Diabetes: Insulin-like proteins found in moringa may help lower blood sugar and plant chemicals found in the leaves might help the body to better process sugar, as well as affect how the body releases insulin.
3. Cancer: There have been some reports that indicate that in lab tests of leaf extracts slowed the growth of pancreatic cancer cells and helped chemotherapy work better. Other lab studies show that moringa leaves, bark, and roots all have anti-cancer effects that might lead to new drugs.
4. Memory: Some experts think the antioxidants and other health-promoting plant chemicals may heal stress and inflammation in the brain.

Moringa (Moringa oleifera), also known as the "Miracle Tree," is packed with nutrients, antioxidants, and medicinal properties. Here's how you can consume it for maximum benefits.

Moringa Tea (Gentle & Soothing)

Ingredients:

- 1 to 2 teaspoons of dried Moringa leaves
- 1 cup of hot water

Instructions:

1. Add the dried leaves to a cup of hot water.
2. Let it steep for 5–10 minutes.
3. Strain and drink.
4. You can add honey, ginger, or lemon for taste.

Best time: In the morning or before meals for energy and digestion support.

Cashew

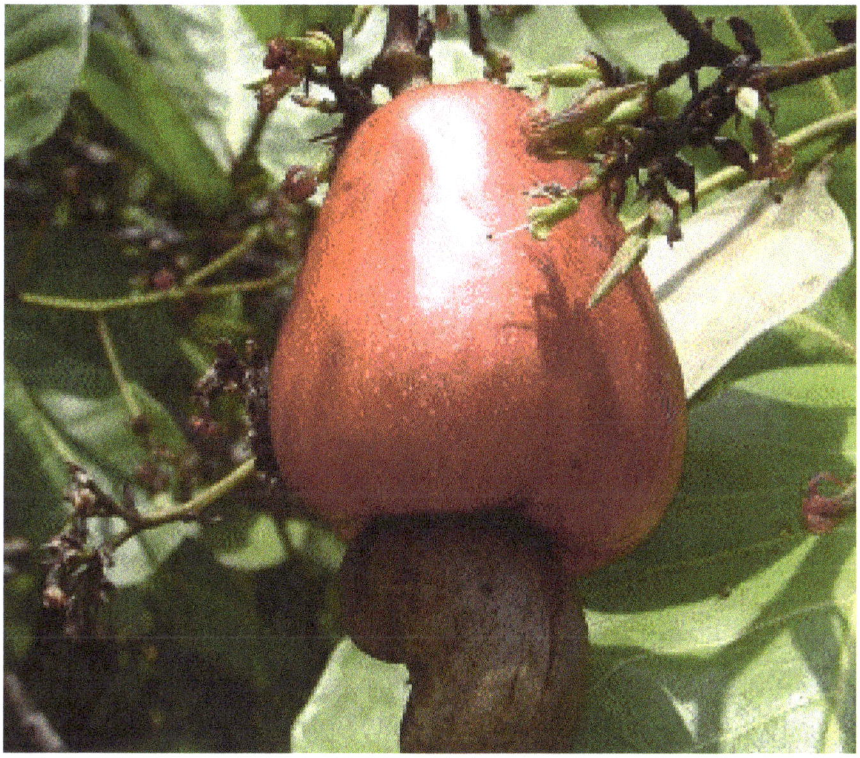

In the Caribbean islands, people eat both the tasty nuts and the 'apple' (or 'banana'), the fleshy structure from which the nut hangs. This is used to make a refreshing drink, wine, brandy and jelly. Its acid, aromatic juice contains five times as much vitamin C as orange juice.

Cashew are very tasty, but they must be roasted before eating, as the thin shell contains a very irritant oil. The active chemicals are cardol and anacardic acid. Roasting gets rid of the oil, but the fumes that arise during roasting can cause skin and eye irritation, inflammation and poisoning.

Every part of the plant appears to have medicinal uses. Jamaican herbalists agree with Sloane that leaf extracts can be used to bathe ulcers or added to baths for fever.
One cold remedy involves a mix of cashew leaves, fern leaves and 'rat ears', wrapped in cashew leaves and then boiled.

An infusion of leaves and bark is used for dysentery, toothache and sore gums.
In the tree's native country, Brazil, bark teas are used for diarrhoea, and the caustic shell oil for skin infections, warts, worms and botfly larvae beneath the skin.

Resins and gums from the bark and stems (cacajou gum) are used in varnishes for books, wood and flooring, to protect from ants and other home-invading insects. The sap is said to have insecticidal properties.

The shell oil is used in industry to make plastics and resins. Cashew-nutshell liquid (CNSL) is also used in brake linings and clutches.
Cashew oil and juice are added to facial peels, scalp conditioners and shampoos.

Extracts from cashew apple and bark are reported to act against bacteria that cause some stomach ulcers. The bark and leaves are both rich in tannins and have anti-inflammatory and astringent properties. Leaf extracts have been shown to be useful against lab-induced diabetes. Nutshells have acids toxic to certain cancers.

Cashew tea is a herbal tea made from cashew leaves or cashew bark, traditionally used for its medicinal properties, including anti-inflammatory, antioxidant, and digestive benefits. Here's how to prepare it:
Cashew Leaf Tea Recipe

Ingredients:

- 5–7 fresh or dried cashew leaves
- 2 cups of water
- Honey or lemon (optional, for taste)

Instructions:

1. Rinse the Leaves: Wash the cashew leaves thoroughly.
2. Boil Water: Bring 2 cups of water to a boil.
3. Add Leaves: Add the cashew leaves and reduce the heat to low.
4. Simmer: Let it simmer for 10–15 minutes to extract the nutrients.
5. Strain & Serve: Remove the leaves, pour the tea into a cup, and enjoy.
6. Optional: Add honey or lemon for flavor.

Best Time to Drink: Morning or before bed for relaxation and digestive support.

Coconut

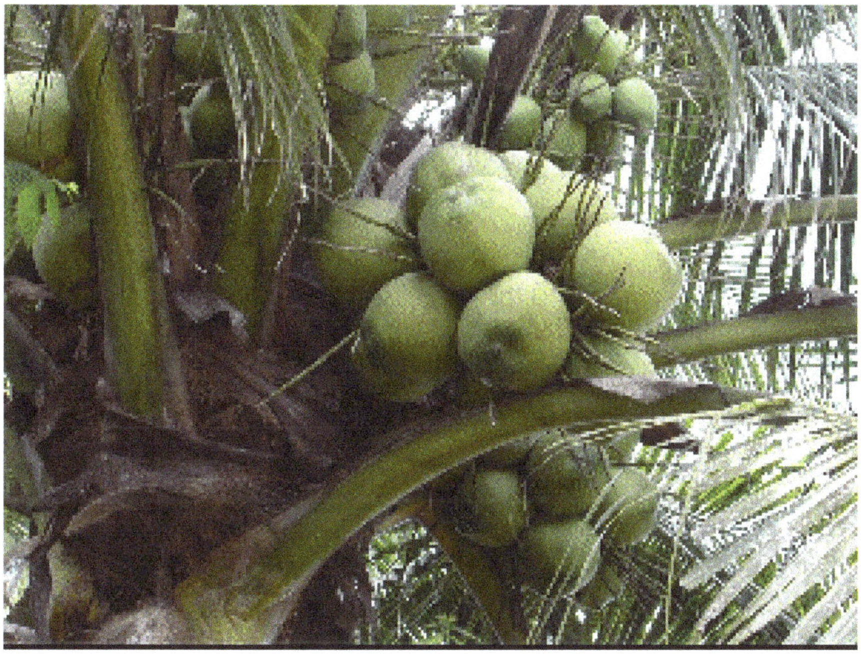

Today, the coconut palm is as valued in the Caribbean as it was 300 years ago. The leaves are used for shelter, the shell for carving, the kernel for food, the oil for medication and cosmetics, and the waste for animal fodder. As a medicine, it is widely seen as good for the heart and digestion. Boiling up young coconuts with white rum, for example, makes a drink to cure stomach upsets and dysentery.

A coconut is in fact a fruit, with a single seed. There are three layers, one made out of a smooth green outer skin, underneath is a fibrous layer of coir, and lastly the hard dark-brown shell of the seed.

Inside, the seed has firm white flesh (copra) and a sweet liquid as milk or water, which thickens with time. Coconut milk used in cooking is the grated white flesh mixed with the water. The flesh is eaten fresh, or dried and pressed to release its oil, which is used in shampoos and hair conditioners.

The coir is used to make matting, and is now an important alternative to peat in compost. The hard shell can be used as a cup or container. Sloane was sceptical about island claims that any liquor drunk out of a coconut shell would gain medicinal properties from it.

Some research suggests coconut oil helps with immune problems. It seems to reduce the amount of virus in the body and therefore might be beneficial to HIV and AIDS patients. It also contains anti-microbial chemicals.

Coconut oil can be consumed in several ways, depending on your health goals and preferences. Here are some common ways to incorporate it into your diet:

1. Direct Consumption

- How? Take 1 teaspoon to 1 tablespoon daily.
- Best for: Boosting metabolism, improving digestion, and increasing energy levels.

Tip: Start with a small amount to avoid stomach discomfort.

2. Cooking and Baking

- How? Use coconut oil instead of butter or vegetable oil for frying, sautéing, roasting, or baking.
- Best for: A healthy alternative in recipes for stir-fries, scrambled eggs, or baked goods.

3. In Beverages

- How? Add 1 teaspoon to 1 tablespoon to coffee, tea, or smoothies.
- Best for: Energy boost and improved mental clarity.
- Blend well to prevent oil separation.

4. With Food

- How? Drizzle over salads, oatmeal, or yogurt.
- Best for: A nutritious addition to meals with a light coconut flavor.

5. As a Supplement

- How? Mix with apple cider vinegar or lemon juice for digestive and immune support.
- Best for: Gut health, weight management, and overall wellness.

Cannabis

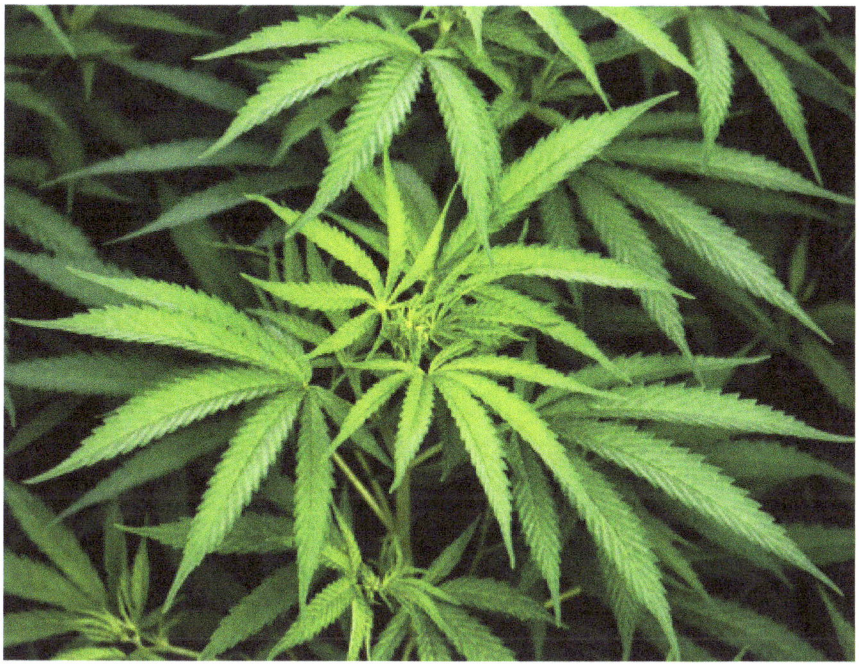

Used worldwide since ancient times as treatment for various conditions and ailments including pain, inflammation, gastrointestinal issues such as IBS, muscle relaxation, anxiety, Alzheimer's and dementia, ADHD, autism, cancer, cerebral palsy, recurring headaches, Crohn's disease, depression, epilepsy, glaucoma, insomnia, and neuropathy among others.

The history of the cannabis plant

The medicinal properties of the cannabis plant have been known for millennia. As far back as 2800 BC, cannabis was used to treat a vast array of health problems and was listed in Emperor Shen Nung's pharmacopoeia.

Cannabis has a long and colourful history. The use of cannabis originated in central Asia or western China. Cannabis has been used for its alleged healing properties for millennia. The first documented case of its use dates back to 2800 BC, when it was listed in the Emperor Shen Nung's (regarded as the father of Chinese medicine) pharmacopoeia.

Therapeutic indications of cannabis are mentioned in the texts of the Indian Hindus, Assyrians, Greeks and Romans. These texts reported cannabis to treat a vast array of different health problems, including arthritis, depression, amenorrhea, inflammation, pain, lack of appetite and asthma.

Hindu legend holds that Shiva, the supreme Godhead of many sects, was given the title 'The Lord of Bhang', because the cannabis plant was his favourite food. The ancient Hindus thought the medicinal benefits of cannabis were explained by pleasing the gods such as Shiva.

Cannabis has various health benefits and can be used in different forms depending on your needs. Below are some common ways to use cannabis for health purposes:

- Inhalation (Smoking or Vaping)
- How? Smoke dried cannabis flowers or use a vaporizer.
- Best for: Immediate relief from pain, anxiety, stress, nausea, and insomnia.
- Vaping is a healthier alternative to smoking as it reduces exposure to harmful toxins.

1. Edibles (Infused Foods & Drinks)

- How? Consume cannabis-infused gummies, chocolates, tea, or oil.
- Best for: Long-lasting relief from chronic pain, inflammation, and sleep disorders.

Tip: Effects take longer (30 minutes to 2 hours) to kick in but last longer than smoking. Start with a low dose.

2. Cannabis Tinctures (Sublingual Use)

- How? Place a few drops of cannabis tincture under your tongue for quick absorption.
- Best for: Quick relief from pain, stress, and anxiety.
- Ideal for those who want precise dosing without smoking.

3. Cannabis Oils & Capsules

- How? Ingest cannabis oil or capsules as a supplement.
- Best for: Managing pain, inflammation, seizures, and improving overall health.

4. Cannabis Tea or Juicing (Raw Cannabis Leaves & Flowers)

- How? Brew raw cannabis leaves into tea or blend into smoothies.
- Best for: Anti-inflammatory effects, digestion, and immune system support.
- Raw cannabis is rich in cannabinoids like THCA and CBDA, which have health benefits without causing a high.

Calabash

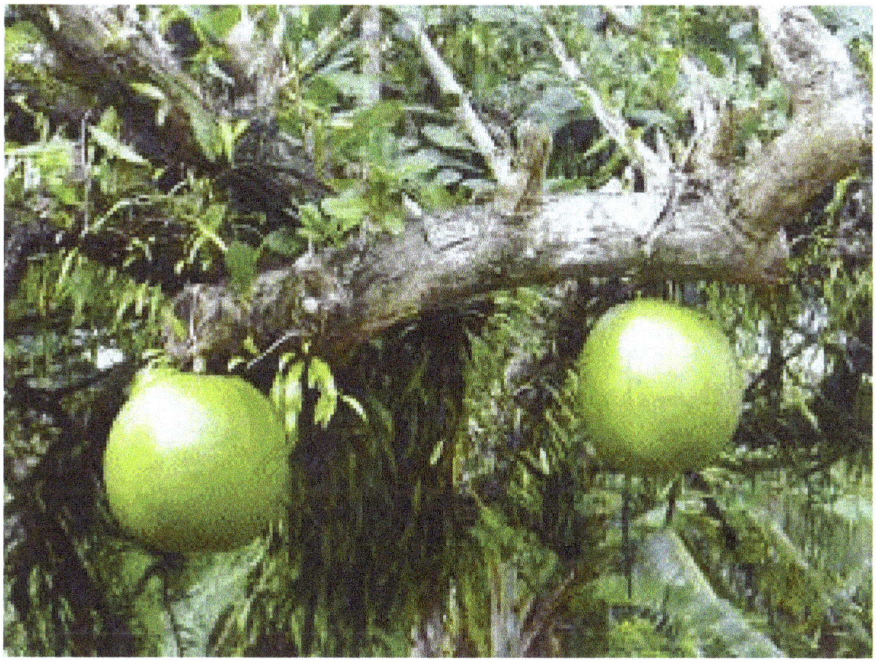

The plant is less well known as a traditional medicine. A drink made from the fruit pulp is still recorded (on islands such as Aruba) as a remedy for colds and flu. The calabash's large hard-cased fruit, known as a gourd, is the most useful part of the tree. Hollowed out, they are made into containers of different sizes, from drinking cups to large bowls.

They are also used for making musical instruments, especially the maracas. The hollow gourds are filled with pebbles or hard seeds that rattle when shaken. Invented by the Taino, they were later taken up by plantation slaves.

Taino hunters cut eye holes in gourds and put them on over their heads before wading into water to hunt birds. The birds saw no danger in what looked like floating gourds, so the hunters could get close enough to catch them.

Calabash (Lagenaria siceraria) is a medicinal plant traditionally used for various health benefits. Here's how it can be used:

Calabash (Lagenaria siceraria) is a medicinal plant traditionally used for various health benefits. Here's how it can be used:

1. Calabash Tea (for Coughs, Asthma, and Respiratory Issues)

How to Make:

- Cut the dried calabash shell into small pieces.
- Boil a handful in 3 cups of water for 10–15 minutes.
- Strain and drink 1 cup daily.

Benefits:

- Helps with asthma and bronchitis.
- Clears mucus and soothes the throat.

2. Calabash Leaves (for Inflammation & Wounds)

How to Use:

- Crush fresh leaves and apply as a poultice to wounds, burns, or swelling.

Benefits:

- Helps with skin infections and inflammation.
- 3. Calabash Fruit Juice (for Digestion & Detoxification)

How to Use:

- Blend fresh calabash pulp with water.
- Drink ½ cup in the morning on an empty stomach.

Benefits:

- Aids digestion and relieves constipation.
- Acts as a natural detoxifier.

3. Calabash Seeds (for Parasites & Liver Health)

How to Use:

- Dry the seeds and grind them into a powder.
- Take ½ teaspoon with warm water before meals.

Benefits:

- Helps eliminate intestinal parasites.
- Supports liver function.

Soursop leaves (Cancer Killer)

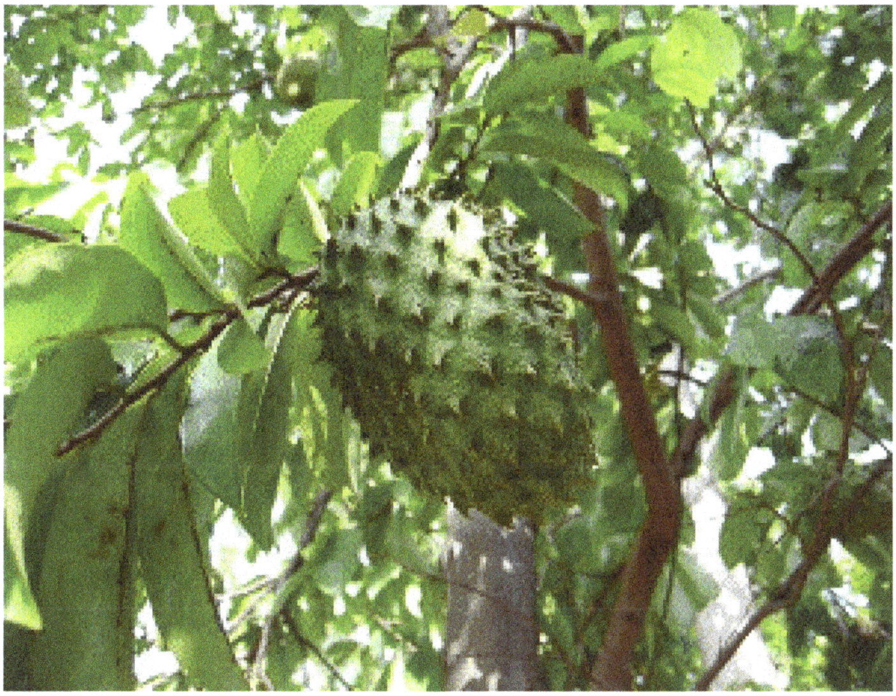

Soursop leaves have an important place in traditional medicine and the Caribbean, Central and South America, although different from the uses Sloane recorded. A tea of the leaves is used to soothe nerves and high blood pressure brought on by them. It's also taken for flu and fevers and a host of digestive problems.

Fresh leaves give a good night's sleep. In the Antilles, they are put into a pillowslip or strewn on the bed, or drunk in tea before bed. Mashed leaves are used to soothe inflammations and heal sores and wounds. And, interestingly, rubbing the head with leaves and water is said to sober up a drunk.

The leathery green fruit of the soursop can be found in markets across the tropics. It has a delicious white creamy pulp with a slight smell of pineapple, and lots of black seeds. Scooped from the rind, the flesh can be eaten fresh, or pulped and turned into icecream. Its creamy juice makes a refreshing drink mixed with sugar and water or milk.
A fermented, cider-like drink is also sometimes made, and unripe, sour fruits can be eaten as vegetables.

An infusion of leaves, some pounded seeds or seed oil, are all said to kill head lice and bedbugs, as well as being a good general pesticide. The bark, seeds and roots have been used as fish poison.

The fruit is typically oval or heart-shaped and can weight up to 6.8 kilogrammes. It's covered with a leathery, inedible bitter skin with stubby, soft, pliable spines. Their tips break off easily when the fruit is fully ripe. The pulp inside may contain 30-200 smooth black-brown seeds, which are slightly toxic.

Chemicals in the leaves, seeds and stem have been shown to kill certain cancer cells, while leaving healthy dividing cells alone. There are also claims of antiviral properties.

How to Make Soursop Leaves Tea

Ingredients:

- 3 to 5 fresh or dried soursop leaves
- 2 cups of water
- Honey or lemon (optional)

Instructions:

- Wash the leaves thoroughly to remove any dirt or residue.
- Boil the water in a pot.
- Add the leaves and let them simmer for 10–15 minutes on low heat.
- Strain the tea into a cup.

Add honey or lemon if desired for taste.
Drink 1–2 cups daily, preferably on an empty stomach or before meals.

Fitweed

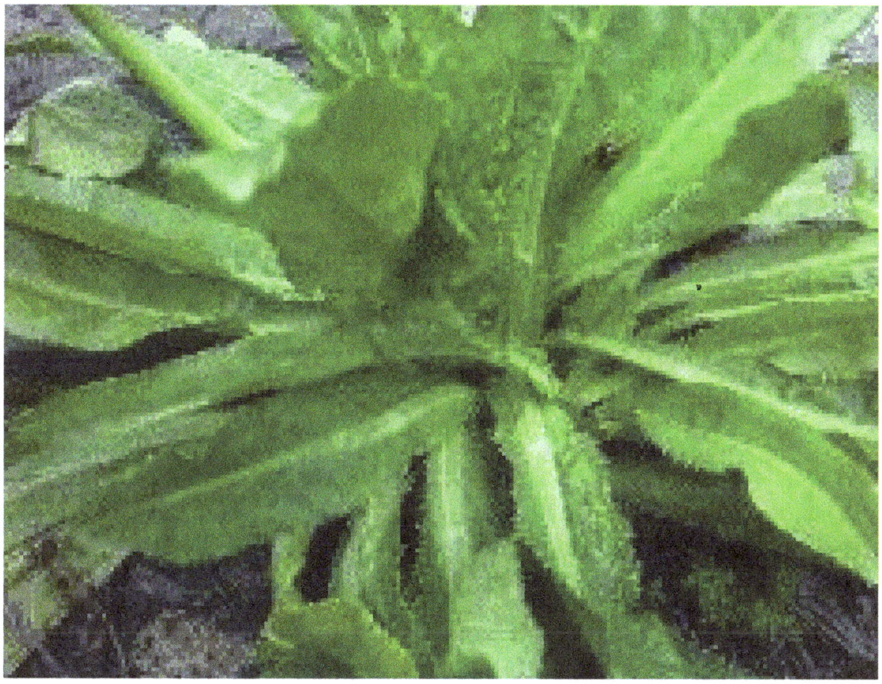

Fitweed is a popular food herbs in the Caribbean. It is one of many 'corianders' used across the world, although it is not closely related. A chutney made with fitweed leaves, they say, stimulates the appetite.

As a medicine, fitweed is recommended in a tea for diarrhoea, vomiting and constipation and also for flu and fevers. In Jamaica it's used for colds and convulsions in children and, combined with Rivina humili (rouge plant), to treat eye diseases. It is also used to bring on menstrual bleeding.

Some herbalists say fitweed is an aphrodisiac and, indeed, Sloane commented it 'excites venery' (sexual intercourse). He also noted its use for venomous snakebites. The root, eaten raw, is said to be good for scorpion stings.

As well as being a popular food herb, it appears in many herbal traditions. In Brazil it's used to bring down fevers, in Africa for headaches and boils.

The plant is said to calm a person's 'spirit' and thus prevents epileptic 'fits', so is known by the common names spiritweed and fitweed.

How to Make Fitweed Tea (Eryngium Foetidum Tea)

Fitweed, also known as Eryngium foetidum, spiny coriander, or shadow beni, is a powerful medicinal herb used for its anti-inflammatory, antioxidant, and digestive benefits. It is commonly used in herbal medicine to treat colds, fevers, and digestive issues.

Ingredients:

- 5–7 fresh fitweed leaves (or 1 teaspoon dried fitweed)
- 2 cups of water
- Honey or lemon (optional, for taste)

Instructions:

1. Wash the Leaves – Rinse the fitweed leaves thoroughly to remove dirt and debris.
2. Boil Water – Bring 2 cups of water to a boil in a pot.
3. Add Fitweed Leaves – Add the fresh or dried fitweed leaves to the boiling water.
4. Simmer – Reduce the heat and let it simmer for 5–10 minutes.
5. Strain – Remove from heat and strain the tea into a cup.
6. Add Sweeteners (Optional) – You can add honey or lemon for flavor.
7. Drink Warm – Enjoy the tea while warm for the best health benefits.

Health Benefits of Fitweed Tea:

✓ Relieves Cold & Flu Symptoms – Helps clear mucus and soothes sore throats.
✓ Supports Digestion – Relieves bloating, gas, and stomach aches.
✓ Reduces Inflammation – Helps with arthritis, joint pain, and swelling.
✓ Promotes Detoxification – Cleanses the liver and kidneys.
✓ Boosts Immunity – Strengthens the body's defense against infections.

Mammee

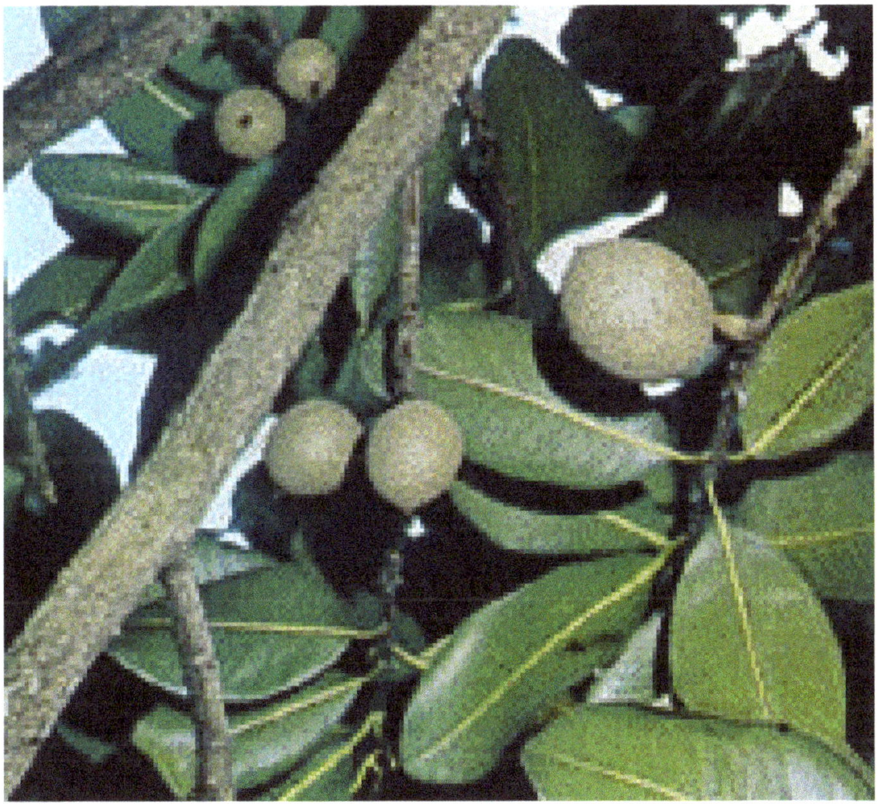

In Jamaica, the mammee bark gum is melted with fat, and smeared onto animals' feet to get rid of fleas and other parasites. Infusions of half-ripe fruits are said to have the same effect.

You can find mammee apples in many Caribbean markets. They are oval, the size of a large orange, with a thick, leathery, bitter skin. Inside, the reddish or yellow flesh is sweet and aromatic, and tastes a bit like apricot.

Mammees are usually eaten raw or stewed and eaten as a dessert. They are also used for jams and preserves, as Sloane recorded.
In French-speaking parts of the Caribbean, people make a liqueur, from the flowers, and also drink it as a tonic.

In Central and Southern America, ground-up mammee seeds stirred into hot water are used to treat parasitic skin diseases and worms.
The leaves are said to contain insecticidal chemicals, and in Puerto Rico farmers wrap them around young tomato plants to keep pests away. The seeds are toxic to fish, chicks and some insects.

Mammee apple (Mammea americana) leaves have been traditionally used in herbal medicine for their potential health benefits. Here are some of the known benefits and ways to use them:

Health Benefits of Mammee Leaves

1. Anti-Inflammatory Properties

- Mammee leaves contain compounds that may help reduce inflammation, making them beneficial for conditions like arthritis and joint pain.

2. Antimicrobial & Antifungal Effects

- Traditionally used to help fight infections, the leaves may have antibacterial and antifungal properties.

3. Supports Digestive Health

- Drinking mammee leaf tea may aid digestion and help with stomach discomfort.

4. **May Support Blood Sugar Control**

- Some traditional uses suggest that mammee leaves can help regulate blood sugar levels.

5. Detoxification & Cleansing

- Mammee leaf tea is sometimes used as a natural detoxifier to help cleanse the body.

Mammee Leaf Tea

How to Make:

- Wash a handful of fresh or dried leaves.
- Boil in 2-3 cups of water for 10-15 minutes.
- Let it cool, strain, and drink warm or chilled.
- Add honey or ginger for taste.

Herbal Bath or Steam Treatment

- Boil the leaves in water and use the steam for skin cleansing.
- Strain the boiled water and add it to a bath for relaxation.

Lavender

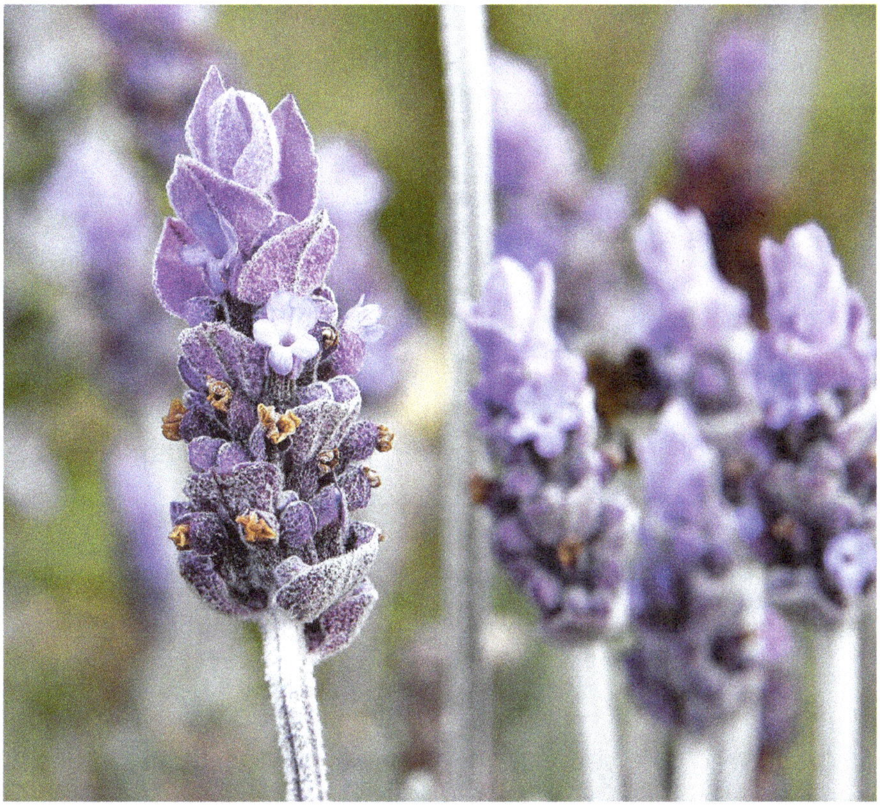

Lavender may have various health benefits, including relieving anxiety and depression and supporting skin health. You can consume it, such as a tea or capsule, apply it topically, or use it for aromathcrapy

Many people appreciate lavender (Lavandula angustifolia or Lavandula officinalis) for its fragrance. Lavendar is a common ingredient in soaps, shampoos, and sachets for scenting clothes.

The name lavender comes from the Latin root lavare, which means "to wash." Lavender may have earned this name because it was frequently used in baths to help purify the body and spirit.

However, this herb has also been used as a remedy for a range of ailments from insomnia and anxiety to depression and fatigue. Research has confirmed that lavender produces slight calming, soothing, and sedative effects when its scent is inhaled.

Medicinal Uses and Indications

A number of studies have reported that lavender essential oil may be beneficial in a variety of conditions, including insomnia, alopecia (hair loss), anxiety, stress, and postoperative pain. However, most of these studies have been small. Lavender is also being studied for antibacterial and antiviral properties.

Lavender oil is often used in other forms of integrative medicine, such as massage, acupuncture, and chiropractic manipulation.

Insomnia or Agitation

In folklore, pillows were filled with lavender flowers to help restless people fall sleep. Scientific evidence suggests that aromatherapy with lavender may slow the activity of the nervous system, improve sleep quality, promote relaxation, and lift mood in people suffering from sleep disorders.

Studies also suggest that massage with essential oils, particularly lavender, may result in improved sleep quality, more stable mood, better concentration, and reduced anxiety.

In one study, people who received massage with lavender felt less anxious and more positive than those who received massage alone. Several small studies suggest that lavender aromatherapy may help reduce agitation in people with dementia.
Lavender flowers have also been approved in Germany as a tea for insomnia, restlessness, and nervous stomach irritations.

Alopecia areata

In one study of 86 people with alopecia areata (an autoimmune disease that causes hair to fall out, often in patches), those who massaged their scalps with lavender and other essential oils daily for 7 months experienced significant hair regrowth compared to those who massaged their scalps without the essential oils.
However, there is no way to tell whether it was one or the combination of oils that was effective. On the other hand, preliminary studies also show that lavendar may be effective in treating women with hirsuitism
(excessive hair growth).

How to Make Lavender Tea for Insomnia

Lavender tea is known for its calming effects and is widely used to promote relaxation, reduce anxiety, and improve sleep quality. Drinking lavender tea before bed can help treat insomnia naturally.

Ingredients:

- 1–2 teaspoons of dried lavender buds (or 2–3 fresh lavender sprigs)
- 1 cup of hot water
- Honey or chamomile (optional, for added relaxation)

Instructions:

1. Boil Water – Heat 1 cup of water until it reaches a gentle boil.
2. Steep Lavender – Place the dried or fresh lavender in a teacup or teapot and pour the hot water over it.
3. Cover and Steep – Let it steep for 5–10 minutes to extract the essential oils.
4. Strain and Serve – Remove the lavender flowers by straining the tea.
5. Sweeten (Optional) – Add honey or mix with chamomile for enhanced relaxation.
6. Drink Warm Before Bed – Consume 30–60 minutes before sleep for best results.

Health Benefits of Lavender Tea for Insomnia:

✓ Promotes Relaxation – Reduces stress and anxiety.
✓ Improves Sleep Quality – Induces drowsiness and enhances deep sleep.
✓ Eases Tension – Soothes headaches and muscle tension.
✓ Calms the Nervous System – Helps with restlessness and nervous exhaustion.

Thyme tea

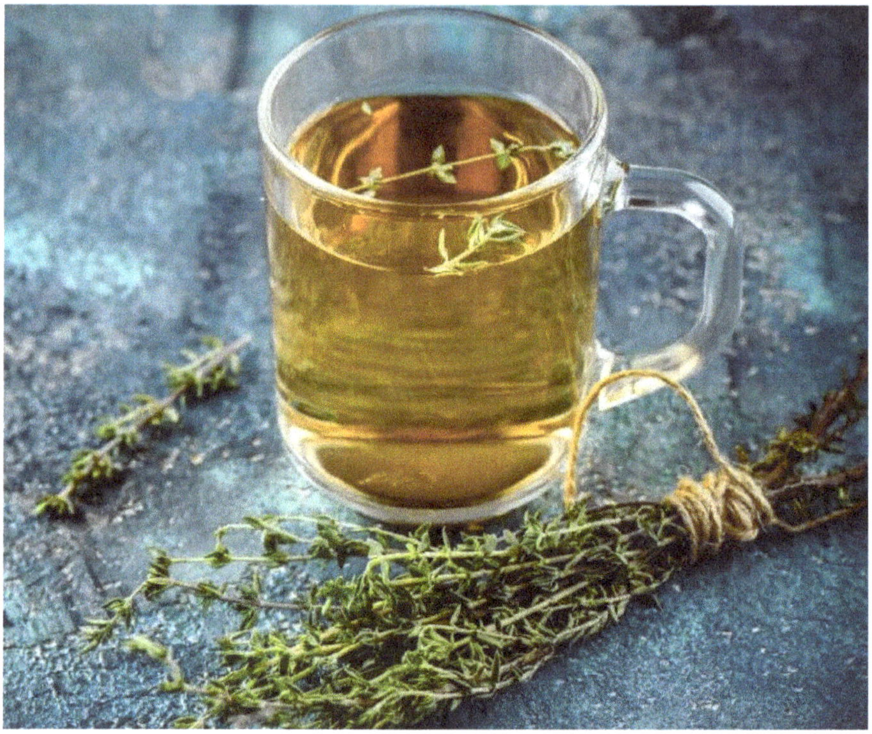

Thyme Tea: A Natural Remedy with Numerous Health Benefits
Thyme tea offers a variety of potential health benefits, including reducing inflammation, improving digestion, and strengthening immunity.

Digestive Health

- May help relieve indigestion and gas discomfort
- Supports healthy digestion

Immune Support

- Packed with essential vitamins and minerals that boost the immune system
- Rich in phenol, a powerful antiseptic

Respiratory Health

- Anti-inflammatory properties may help ease respiratory issues like coughing and nasal congestion can provide relief from colds, flu, and tonsillitis

Stress Relief

- Has a calming effect that may help reduce stress and anxiety

Skin Health

- High in antioxidants, which promote healthy skin
- Antibacterial properties may help combat mild acne and skin congestion

Other Potential Benefits

May help lower blood pressure

- Could provide relief from menstrual pain
- May aid in weight management
- Supports natural detoxification
- May promote better sleep
-
- Thyme tea is a soothing herbal infusion made from the leaves of the thyme plant, a versatile perennial herb. Beyond tea, thyme is commonly used as a seasoning for meats, fish, vegetables, sauces, pasta, and soups.
- This version keeps everything organized while making sure lower blood pressure is included.

Here's a simple and effective way to make thyme tea, a wonderful herbal remedy known for its antiviral, antibacterial, and respiratory-supporting properties.

How to Make Thyme Tea

Ingredients:

- 1–2 teaspoons of fresh or dried thyme leaves
- 1 cup of boiling water
- Optional: lemon, honey, or a pinch of ginger for added benefits and taste

Instructions:

1. Rinse fresh thyme leaves if using.
2. Place the thyme (fresh or dried) in a cup or teapot.
3. Pour 1 cup of boiling water over the thyme.
4. Cover and let it steep for 5–10 minutes.
5. Strain the tea into your cup.
6. Add honey and lemon if desired.

Garlic

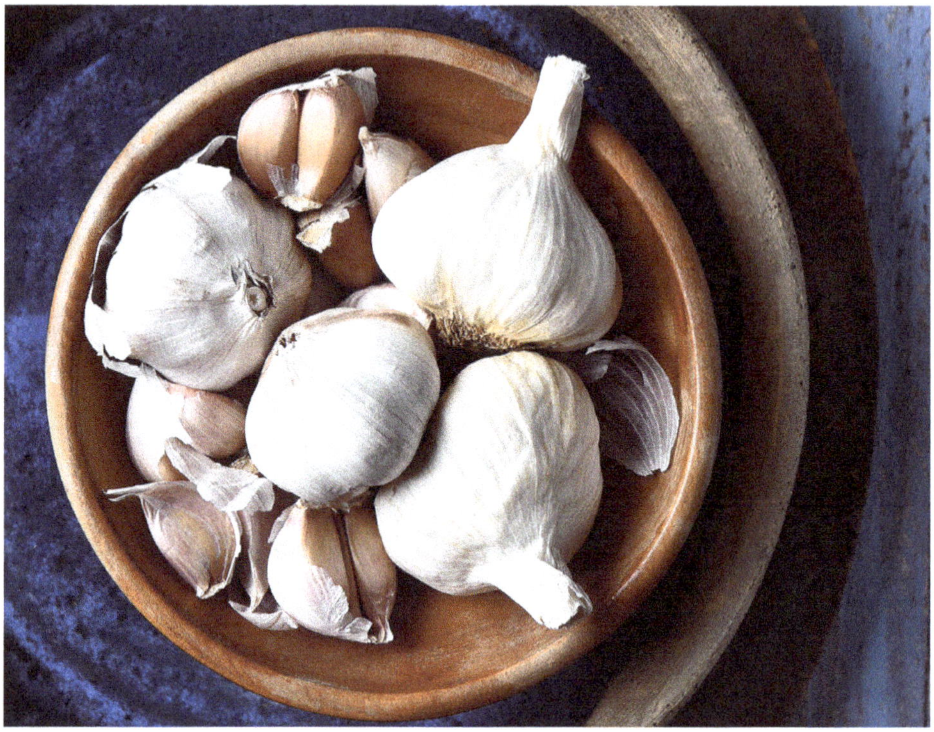

Current research shows that garlic may have some real health benefits, such as protection against the common cold and the ability to help lower blood pressure and cholesterol levels.

Garlic is a plant in the Allium (onion) family. It's closely related to onions, shallots, and leeks. Each segment of a garlic bulb is called a clove. There are about 10–20 cloves in a single bulb, give or take. Garlic grows in many parts of the world and is a popular ingredient in cooking due to its strong smell and delicious taste.

However, throughout ancient history, people widely used garlic for its health and medicinal properties. There is documented evidence of its use by many major civilizations, including the Egyptians, Greeks, Romans, Chinese, and Indians.

Scientists now know that most of garlic's health benefits are due to the formation of sulfur compounds when you chop, crush, or chew a garlic clove.
Perhaps the most well-known compound is allicin. However, allicin is an unstable compound that is only briefly present in fresh garlic after you cut or crush it.

Ways to Consume Garlic for Health Benefits

1. Raw Garlic (Best for Maximum Benefits)

- Crush or chop 1-2 cloves and let it sit for 10 minutes to activate allicin (the key healing compound).
- Swallow with water or mix with honey for better taste.

2. Garlic & Honey (For Immunity Boost)

- Chop fresh garlic and mix with raw honey.
- Take 1 teaspoon daily on an empty stomach.

3. Garlic Tea (For Colds & Detox)

- Boil 2-3 crushed garlic cloves in 2 cups of water.
- Add lemon and honey for taste.
- Drink warm to soothe the throat and boost immunity.

4. Garlic Milk (For Digestion & Respiratory Health)

- Boil 3-4 cloves in a cup of milk.
- Drink warm before bed for cough relief and digestion.

5. Garlic & Apple Cider Vinegar (For Blood Pressure & Heart Health)

- Mix crushed garlic with apple cider vinegar and warm water.
- Drink in the morning for heart and blood pressure support.

Onions

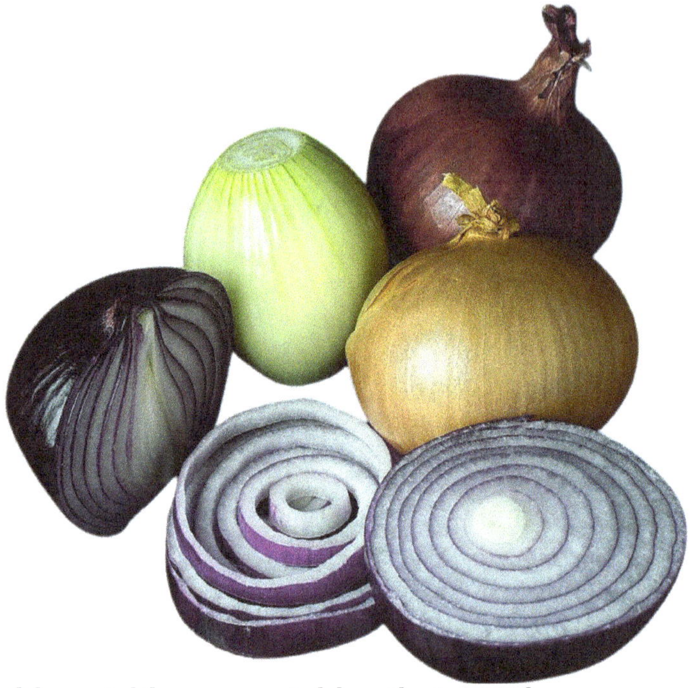

Onions are highly nutritious vegetables that may have several benefits, including improved heart health, better blood sugar regulation, and increased bone density.

Onions are members of the Allium genus of flowering plants, which also includes garlic, shallots, and leeks.They're delicious, versatile, and relatively cheap, and they boast a wide range of healthy vitamins, minerals, and plant compounds.

The medicinal properties of onions have been recognized for thousands of years. Athletes in ancient Greece supposedly used onions to purify their blood, while medieval and traditional doctors prescribed them to help treat headaches, heart disease, and mouth sores.

How to Consume Onions for Health Benefits

Onions are packed with antioxidants, vitamins, and sulfur compounds that provide numerous health benefits, including boosting immunity, improving heart health, and reducing inflammation. Here are different ways to consume onions for maximum health benefits:

1. Raw Consumption (Best for Nutrient Retention)

- Eat raw onion slices in salads, sandwiches, or as a side dish.
- Make onion juice by blending raw onions with a little water and drinking a tablespoon daily for detoxification and immunity.

2. Onion Tea (For Cold & Flu Relief)

- Boil 1 chopped onion in 2 cups of water for 10 minutes.
- Strain, add honey and lemon, and drink warm.

3. Onion Infused Honey (For Cough & Sore Throat)

- Chop onions and soak them in raw honey for 12–24 hours.
- Take a spoonful as a natural cough syrup.

4. Onion Soup (For Heart Health & Immunity Boosting)

Prepare a homemade onion and garlic soup with turmeric and black pepper for anti-inflammatory benefits.

5. Fermented Onions (For Gut Health)

Soak chopped onions in apple cider vinegar for 24 hours and consume as a probiotic-rich condiment.

6. Onion Water (For Detox & Blood Sugar Control)

Soak sliced onions in water overnight and drink the infused water in the morning.

Health Benefits of Onions

✓ Boosts Immunity – Rich in antioxidants and vitamin C.
✓ Improves Digestion – Contains prebiotic fiber that supports gut health.
✓ Lowers Blood Pressure – Contains quercetin, which helps regulate blood pressure.
✓ Reduces Inflammation – Helps with joint pain and respiratory issues.
✓ Supports Heart Health – Reduces cholesterol and improves circulation.

Ginger

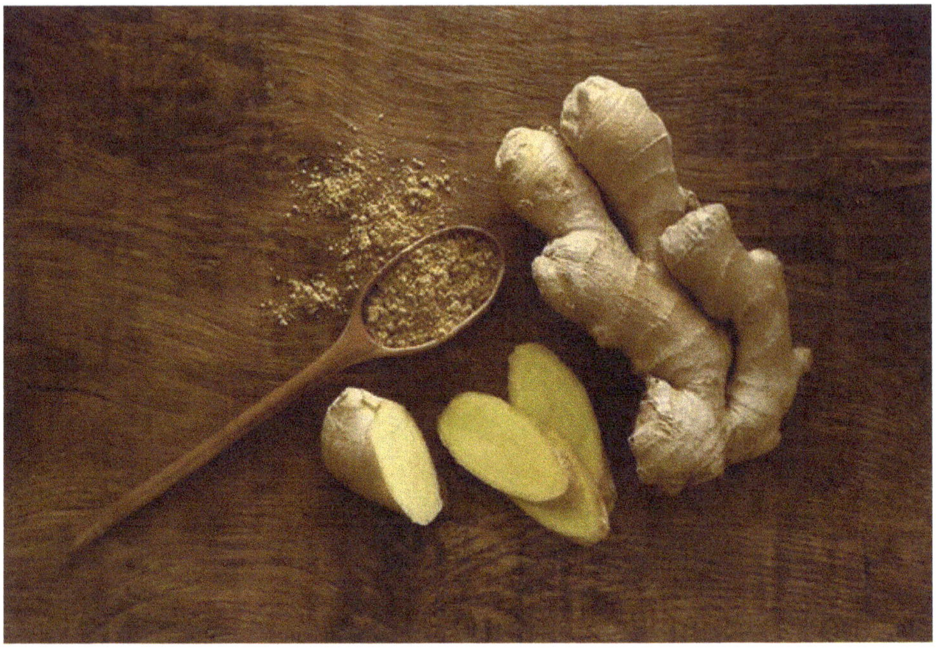

What is ginger good for?

In addition to great taste, ginger provides a range of health benefits that you can enjoy in many forms. Here's what you should know about all the ways ginger can add flavor to your food and support your well-being.

Health Benefits of Ginger

Ginger is not just delicious. Gingerol, a natural component of ginger root, benefits gastrointestinal motility — the rate at which food exits the stomach and continues along the digestive process. Eating ginger encourages efficient digestion, so food doesn't linger as long in the gut.

Nausea relief. Encouraging stomach emptying can relieve the discomforts of

nausea due to:

Chemotherapy. Experts who work with patients receiving chemo for cancer, say ginger may take the edge off post-treatment nausea, and without some of the side effects of anti-nausea medications.

Pregnancy. For generations, women have praised the power of ginger to ease "morning sickness" and other queasiness associated with pregnancy. Even the American Academy of Obstetrics and Gynecology mentions ginger as an acceptable nonpharmaceutical remedy for nausea and vomiting.

.

Bloating and gas. Eating ginger can cut down on fermentation, constipation and other causes of bloating and intestinal gas.
Wear and tear on cells. Ginger contains antioxidants. These molecules help manage free radicals, which are compounds that can damage cells when their numbers grow too high.

Is ginger anti-inflammatory? It is possible. Ginger contains over 400 natural compounds, and some of these are anti-inflammatory. More studies will help us determine if eating ginger has any impact on conditions such as rheumatoid arthritis or respiratory inflammation.

Ginger Tea Benefits

Ginger tea is fantastic in cold months, and delicious after dinner. You can add a little lemon or lime, and a small amount of honey and make a great beverage.
Commercial ginger tea bags are available at many grocery stores and contain dry ginger, sometimes in combination with other ingredients.

These tea bags store well and are convenient to brew. Fresh ginger has strong health benefits comparable to those of dried, but tea made with dried ginger may have a milder flavor.
Making ginger root tea with fresh ginger takes a little more preparation but tends to deliver a more intense, lively brew.

How to Make Ginger Tea

It's easy:

- Buy a piece of fresh ginger.
- Trim off the tough knots and dry ends.
- Carefully peel it.
- Cut it into thin, crosswise slices.
- Put a few of the slices in a cup or mug.
- Pour in boiling water and cover.
- To get all the goodness of the ginger, let the slices steep for at least 10 minutes.

Ginger and Garlic Tea

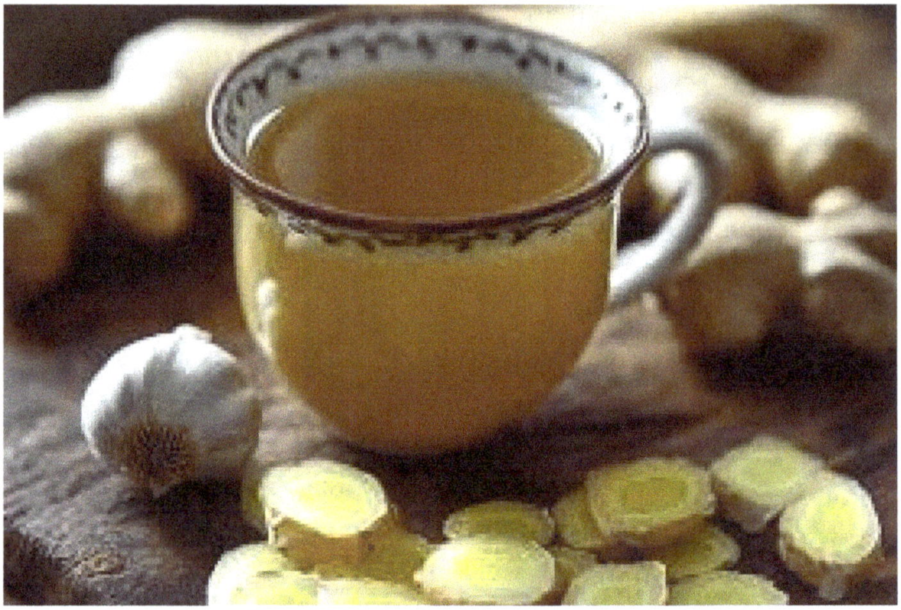

Health Benefits of Ginger and Garlic Tea

Ginger and garlic tea is a powerful herbal infusion with numerous health benefits. Both ingredients contain potent antioxidants, anti-inflammatory compounds, and immune-boosting properties.

1. Boosts Immunity

- Rich in antioxidants that help strengthen the immune system
- Helps fight off colds, flu, and infections

2. Supports Heart Health

- May help lower blood pressure
- Aids in reducing cholesterol levels
- Supports healthy circulation and reduces the risk of heart disease.

3. Aids Digestion

- Helps relieve bloating, indigestion, and gas
- Stimulates the digestive system for better nutrient absorption
- May help alleviate nausea and motion sickness

4. Anti-Inflammatory Properties

- Reduces inflammation and joint pain
- May help relieve arthritis symptoms
- Supports overall body healing.

5. Improves Respiratory Health

Helps clear mucus and ease congestion

May provide relief from sore throat, cough, and bronchitis

Supports lung function and breathing

How to Make Ginger and Garlic Tea

Ingredients:

- 1-inch piece of fresh ginger (or ½ teaspoon powdered ginger)
- 2 cloves of fresh garlic (crushed)
- 2 cups of water
- 1 teaspoon honey (optional)
- ½ teaspoon lemon juice (optional)

Instructions:

1. Peel and slice the ginger into small pieces.
2. Crush the garlic to release its beneficial compounds.
3. Bring the water to a boil in a pot.
4. Add ginger and garlic, then simmer for 10–15 minutes.
5. Strain the tea into a cup.
6. Add honey or lemon for taste (optional).
7. Drink 1–2 cups daily for best results.

Periwinkle

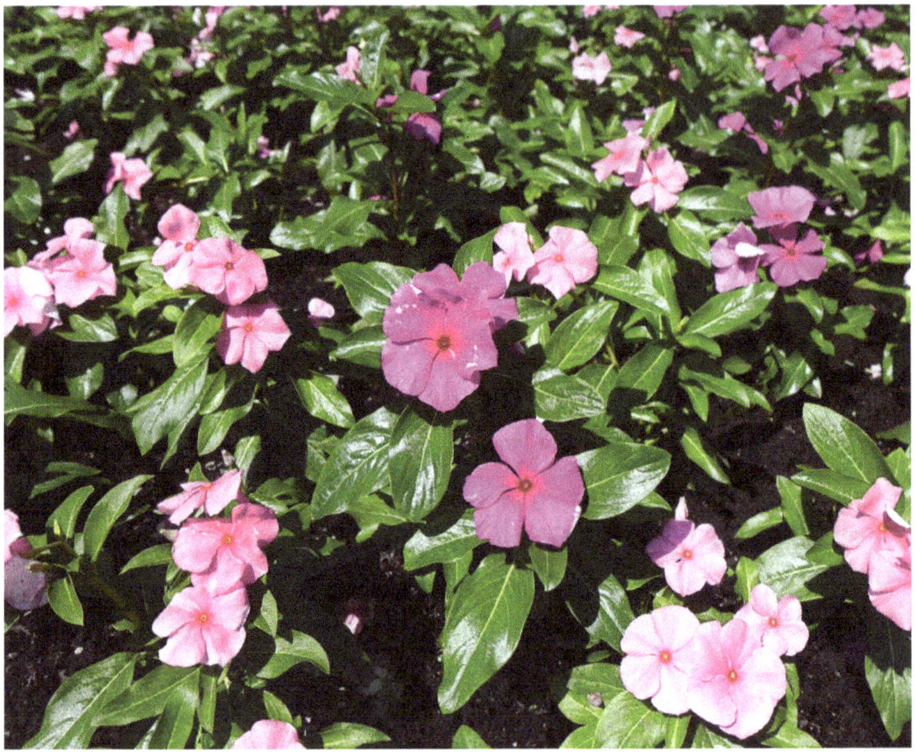

The plant was introduced in Europe during the mid-1700s, during which time it was cultivated as an ornamental. Today it grows throughout much of the world and plantations have been established on most continents in the warmer climates. The plant has been widely used in tropical folk medicine.

Decoctions of the plant have been used for maladies ranging from ocular inflammation, diabetes, and hemorrhage to treating insect stings and cancers.

Miscellaneous uses

Periwinkle alkaloids have been used in the treatment of leukemia, Hodgkin disease, malignant lymphomas, neuroblastoma, Wilms tumor, Kaposi sarcoma, mycosis fungoides, to improve cerebral blood flow, and treat high blood pressure.

The most well known of the "vinca" alkaloids derived from C.

roseus are vinblastine (vincaleukoblastine, Velban) and vincristine (leurocristine, Oncovin), which are now widely used pharmaceutical anticancer agents.

An extensive body of literature exists on the clinical uses of the various purify alkaloids of Catharanthus.

What is the recommended dosage?

There is no recent clinical evidence to support specific doses of periwinkle herb.

Health Benefits of Periwinkle Tea

1. Supports Brain Function & Memory

- Contains vincamine, a compound used in memory-enhancing supplements.
- May help improve focus, concentration, and cognitive function.
- Some studies suggest it may aid in Alzheimer's and dementia prevention.

2. Improves Blood Circulation

- Helps dilate blood vessels, promoting better circulation.
- May help reduce high blood pressure and improve heart health.

3. Natural Stress Reliever & Mood Booster

- May help reduce anxiety and stress due to its calming effects.
- Some herbalists use periwinkle tea to promote emotional balance.

4. Controls Blood Sugar Levels

- Traditionally used to help manage diabetes by regulating blood sugar.
- Helps improve insulin sensitivity.

5. Supports Wound Healing & Skin Health

- Contains antibacterial and anti-inflammatory properties.
- May be applied topically (as a cooled tea wash) to help with wounds, cuts, or rashes.

6. May Help Reduce Headaches & Dizziness

- By improving oxygen flow to the brain, it can help relieve headaches and vertigo.

How to Make Periwinkle Tea

Ingredients:

- 1 teaspoon of dried periwinkle leaves or flowers (or 3 fresh leaves)
- 1 cup of hot water
- Honey or lemon (optional)

Instructions:

1. Boil the water and pour it over the periwinkle leaves.
2. Let it steep for 10–15 minutes.
3. Strain the tea into a cup.
4. Add honey or lemon if desired.
5. Drink 1 cup per day for best results.

Precautions

Do not consume in excess, as high doses can be toxic.

Not recommended for pregnant or breastfeeding women.

People with low blood pressure should consult a doctor before use.

If you are on blood-thinning or diabetes medication, check with your doctor.

Turmeric

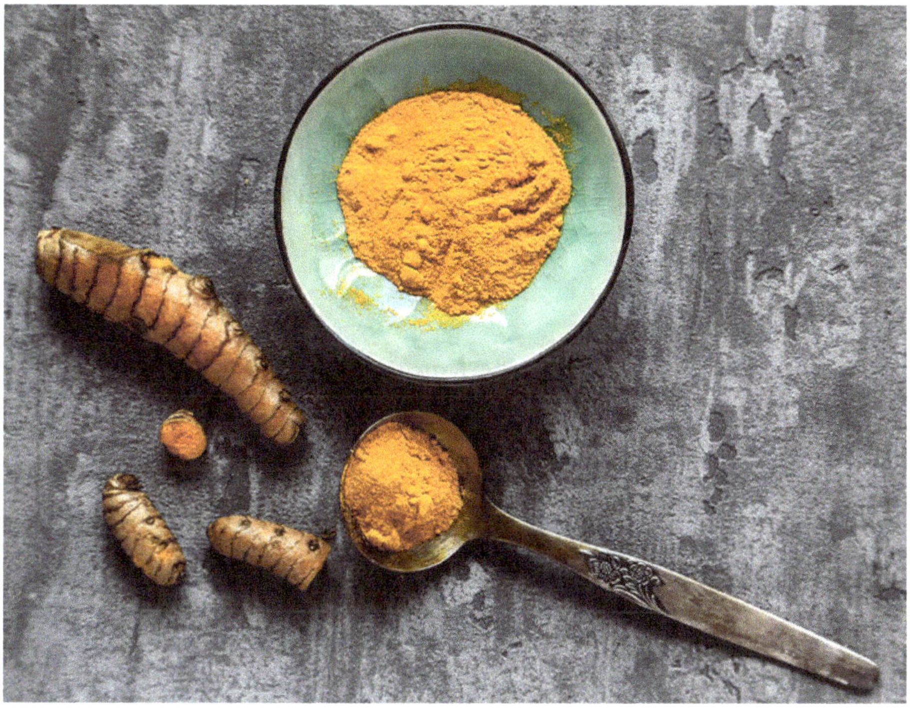

Turmeric's health benefits

Turmeric has been used for thousands of years in Ayurvedic medicine and traditional Chinese medicine to treat conditions such as skin disorders, respiratory problems, joint pain relief, and digestive disorders. More recently, turmeric has become a popular dietary supplement promoted to benefit a variety of conditions including arthritis, digestive disorders, depression, and allergies, among others.

Turmeric has been studied over the past few decades to understand its potential health benefits. One 2020 study found Curcuma to be associated with anti-inflammatory, anticancer, antidiabetic, antidiarrheal, antimicrobial, antiviral, and antioxidant properties.

Research has started to show connections between some of these properties and actual health benefits in people. For example, human studies have shown potential for curcumin in managing osteoarthritis pain. More research is needed to better understand other potential benefits of turmeric, as well as the dosage needed to achieve those benefits.

Incorporating turmeric into your diet

You can incorporate turmeric into your diet by using the spice as a flavoring for many foods and beverages. Turmeric is widely used in Indian cuisine, particularly in curries. It's what gives curries their intense yellow color.

Incorporating turmeric into a meal with fats such as oils can increase the absorption of curcumin by the gastrointestinal tract.

You can also add curcumin as a flavoring to a variety of foods and beverages. For

example:

1.coffee or tea
2.golden milk (combine 1 to 2 teaspoons of turmeric with 1 cup of warm milk, black pepper, cinnamon, and honey or maple syrup over low heat for about 10 minutes.)
3.soups and broths
4.roasted vegetables
5.rice dishes
6.lentil or bean stews.

Guava Leaves Tea

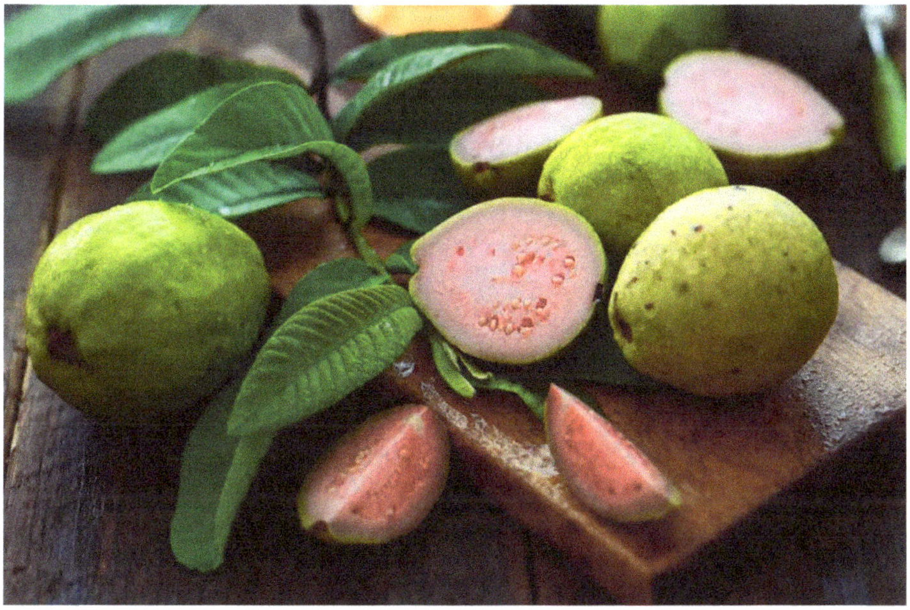

Guava leaf tea has many potential health benefits, including improved blood sugar control, heart health, and digestion. It's also used as a traditional remedy for diarrhea.

Blood sugar

- Guava leaf tea may help regulate blood sugar levels and improve insulin resistance
- It may help suppress blood sugar spikes after eating
- It may be beneficial for people with diabetes or those at risk

Heart health

- Guava leaf tea may help lower blood pressure and reduce LDL cholesterol
- It may help increase HDL cholesterol
- It may help protect the heart from damage by free radicals

Digestion

- Guava leaf tea may help promote gut health
- It may help treat diarrhea

Other benefits

- It may help reduce menstrual cramps
- It may help boost the immune system
- It may help with weight loss

How to Make Guava Leaf Tea

Guava leaf tea is packed with antioxidants, vitamins, and anti-inflammatory compounds. It is commonly used to aid digestion, lower blood sugar levels, support heart health, and boost immunity.

Ingredients:

- 5–7 fresh or dried guava leaves
- 2 cups of water
- 1 teaspoon of honey (optional)
- ½ teaspoon of lemon juice (optional)

Instructions:

1. Wash the Leaves: If using fresh guava leaves, rinse them thoroughly under running water to remove any dirt or chemicals.
2. Boil the Water: In a pot, bring 2 cups of water to a boil.
3. Add the Leaves: Once the water reaches a boil, add the guava leaves.
4. Simmer: Reduce the heat and let it simmer for about 10–15 minutes to allow the nutrients to infuse into the water.
5. Strain the Tea: Remove the pot from heat and strain the tea into a cup.
6. Add Sweeteners (Optional): Add honey or lemon juice for extra flavor.
7. Enjoy: Drink warm for the best results.
8. Health Benefits of Guava Leaf Tea

✔ **Aids Digestion** – Helps with bloating, diarrhea, and stomach discomfort.
✔ **Regulates Blood Sugar** – May lower glucose levels, beneficial for diabetics.
✔ **Boosts Immunity** – High in antioxidants that fight infections.
✔ **Promotes Heart Health** – Helps lower bad cholesterol and improve circulation.
✔ **Supports Weight Loss** – Enhances metabolism and reduces fat absorption.

Castor Oil

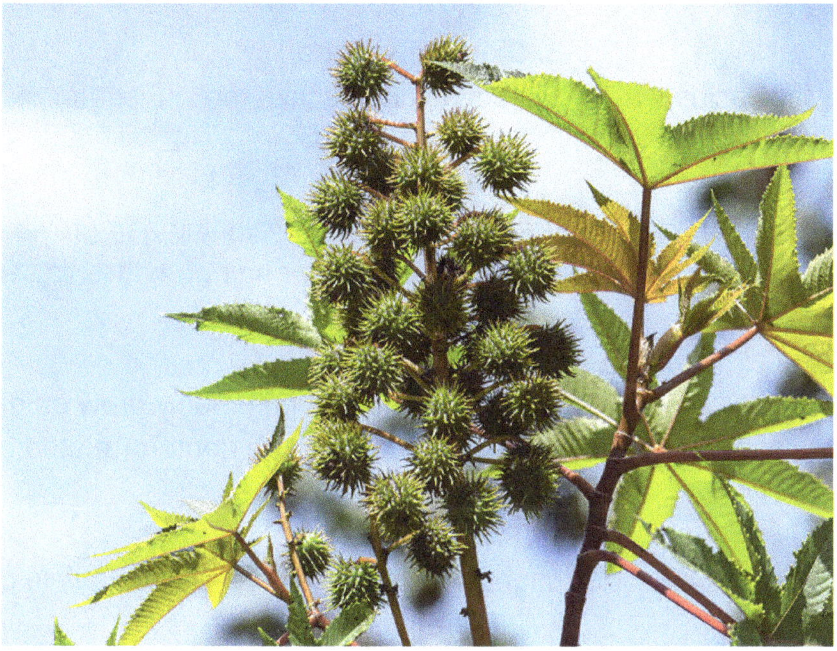

Castor oil is a vegetable oil that people use for various cosmetic and medical purposes. It may provide health benefits for the face and skin, including helping manage acne, moisturizing, and reducing inflammation.

Castor oil, obtained from the Ricinus communis plant, has been used for thousands of years for its remarkable health benefits. This versatile oil offers numerous advantages for everyday use.

Here are 15 essential health benefits of castor oil:

1. Natural Laxative:

The FDA has approved castor oil as a stimulative laxative for the temporary relief of occasional constipation. It works by activating receptors in the intestine, causing muscle contractions.

2. Bowel Preparation:

Castor oil helps in medical procedures like colonoscopies by cleansing the bowel effectively.

3. Anti-inflammatory Characteristics:

The ricinoleic acid in castor oil has anti- inflammatory effects, potentially helping with conditions like arthritis.

4. Antimicrobial Action:
The oil has antibacterial and antimicrobial properties, which may help fight infections.

5. Skin Moisturiser:
Rich in fatty acids, castor oil acts as an effective moisturiser for skin care.

6. Hair Care:
Some people use castor oil for natural hair treatment, including hair growth, dry scalp, and dandruff. However, scientific evidence for hair growth is limited.

7. Denture Care:
Castor oil may help combat fungi like Candida that commonly grow on dentures. This property makes this versatile oil helpful in preventing denture-related oral issues.

8. **Pain Relief:**
When applied topically, castor oil might help alleviate pain, particularly in cases like knee arthritis.

9. **Induce Labour**:
Traditionally, castor oil has been used to aid uterine contractions, though this use isn't FDA-approved.

10. **Digestive Health**: Beyond its laxative effects, castor oil might support overall digestive health.

13. **Immune Support**: Some studies suggest castor oil may have immune-boosting properties.

14. **Industrial and Pharmaceutical Uses**: Castor oil is used in various industries, including as a lubricant and pharmaceuticals.

15. **Potential Acne Treatment**: While not scientifically proven, some people use castor oil to combat acne due to its antibacterial properties.

Other Uses

- Joint/muscle pain: Rub it on sore areas and cover with a warm compress for natural relief.
- Cracked heels: Slather on at night and wear socks to bed.
- Eczema/psoriasis: Helps soothe inflammation and itching—apply gently to affected areas.

Burdock root

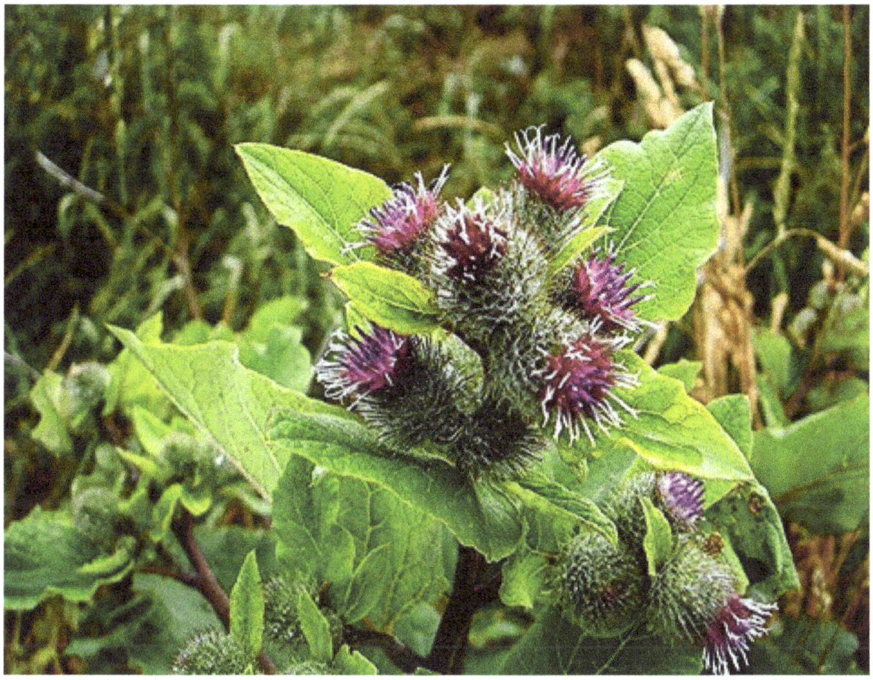

Burdock root has many potential health benefits, including:
Antioxidants: Burdock root contains antioxidants that help protect cells from damage.

- **Anti-inflammatory**: Burdock root can help reduce inflammation, which may help reduce the risk of chronic diseases like diabetes and high blood pressure.
- **Digestion**: Burdock root contains inulin, a natural fiber that improves digestion and gut health.
- **Hair health**: Burdock root contains fiber, essential fatty acids, and vitamins that can help with dry scalp and hair loss.
- **Skin conditions**: Burdock root has been used topically to treat eczema, psoriasis, and other skin conditions.
- **Wound healing**: Burdock root may help wounds heal faster.
- **Blood pressure**: Burdock root may help lower blood pressure.
- **Cancer**: Burdock root has been used in traditional herbal medicine to treat cancer, but more research is needed

Burdock root is a versatile herb known for its detoxifying, anti-inflammatory, and antioxidant properties. You can use it in several ways depending on your goal—whether it's for health, skincare, or cooking. Here's a breakdown of how to use burdock root:

For Health (Internal Use)

1. Burdock Root Tea

- Ingredients: 1–2 teaspoons dried burdock root, 1 cup water.

Instructions:

1. Boil the water and pour it over the dried root.
2. Let it steep for 10–15 minutes.
3. Strain and drink 1–2 cups per day.
4. Benefits: Great for liver health, digestion, and cleansing the blood.

2. Decoction (Stronger than tea)

- Ingredients: 1 tablespoon chopped fresh or dried root, 2 cups water.

Instructions:

1. Simmer for 20–30 minutes.
2. Strain and drink up to twice a day.
3. Use: For more intense detox, skin issues, or as a general tonic.

For Skin (External Use)

1. Burdock Root Infused Oil

- Use: Helps with eczema, acne, psoriasis.

How to make:

- Soak dried burdock root in a carrier oil (like olive or coconut) for 2–4 weeks in a jar. Strain and use on skin or scalp.

Basil

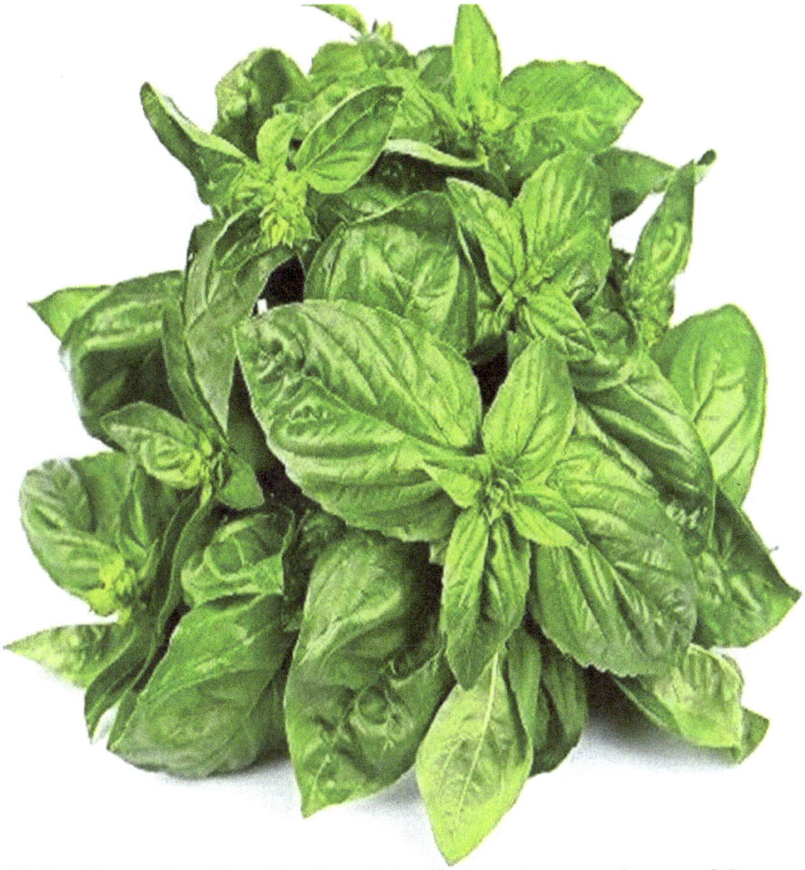

Basil is an herb in the mint family. It adds flavor to meals, and its nutrients may provide health benefits, such as reducing oxidative stress and supporting cardiovascular health.

Sweet basil (Ocimum basilicum) plays a role in many Mediterranean, and particularly Italian, cuisines. It forms the basis of pesto and adds a distinctive flavor to salads, pasta, pizza, and other dishes. Indonesian, Thai, and Vietnamese cuisines also feature this herb.

In the diet, sweet basil can provide vitamins, minerals, and a range of antioxidants. Its essential oil may also have medicinal benefits.
Sweet basil is available in many grocery stores, while other varieties have different tastes and fragrances.

Another type of basil is tulsi, or holy basil (Ocimum santum). This plant plays a therapeutic role in Tamil and Ayurvedic medicines, which are predominantly practiced in Southeast Asia. This is different from sweet basil.

How to Make Basil Tea

Basil tea is a soothing herbal drink known for its antioxidant, anti-inflammatory, and digestive benefits. Here's how you can make it:

Ingredients:

- 1 cup of fresh basil leaves (or 1 tablespoon of dried basil)
- 2 cups of water
- 1 teaspoon of honey or lemon (optional, for flavor)

Instructions:

1. Boil the Water – Bring 2 cups of water to a boil in a pot or kettle.
2. Add the Basil – Turn off the heat and add fresh or dried basil leaves.
3. Steep – Cover and let it steep for 5 to 10 minutes (the longer, the stronger the flavor).
4. Strain & Serve – Strain out the leaves and pour the tea into a cup.
5. Enhance the Flavor – **Add honey, lemon, or ginger for extra benefits and taste.**

Benefits of Basil Tea:

✔ Aids digestion and reduces bloating
✔ Helps relieve stress and anxiety
✔ Supports respiratory health
✔ Boosts immunity

Bilberry

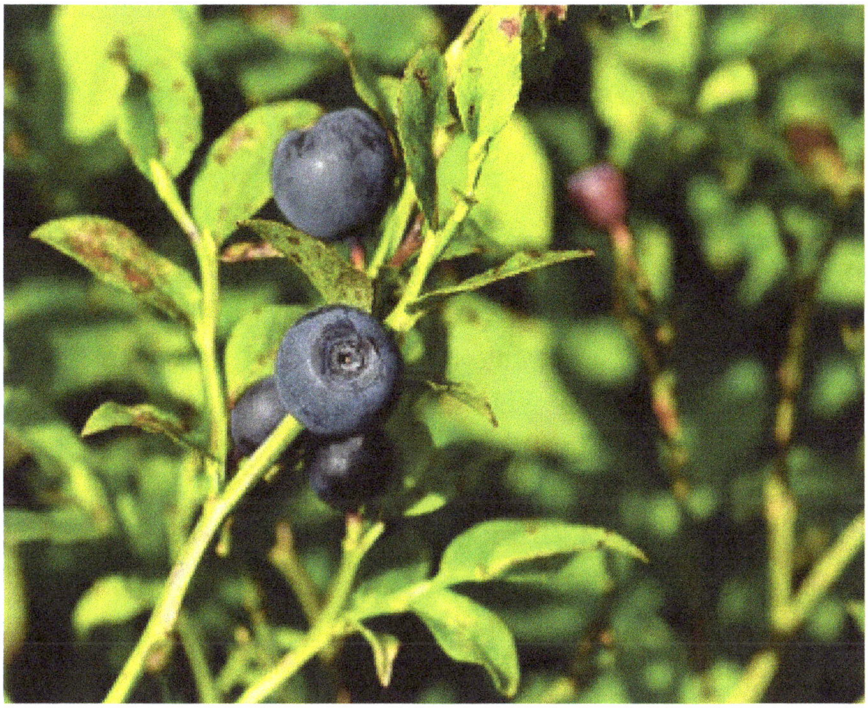

Oh yes—bilberry is one of nature's hidden gems. Think of it as blueberry's wilder, darker, more powerful cousin. It's been used in traditional medicine for centuries, especially for eye health, circulation, and even blood sugar balance.

Health Benefits

Like other types of berries, bilberries have many health benefits. Bilberries contain several plant compounds that can help fight inflammation, improve heart health, prevent diabetes, reduce the risk of cancer, and more.

The health benefits of bilberries include:

Eye health. If left untreated, glaucoma can eventually lead to a gradual loss of eyesight. The anthocyanins in bilberries can help improve eye function for people with normal-tension glaucoma. Some studies suggest bilberries may help with eye fatigue, which can lead to eye strain, headaches, shoulder tension, and blurred or double vision.

Reduced risk of diabetes

Bilberry and bilberry extract can help lower blood sugar levels in people with diabetes. The berries may also help increase insulin secretion in people with metabolic syndrome.

How to Consume Bilberries for Health Benefits

Bilberries are packed with antioxidants, vitamins, and anti-inflammatory properties that support eye health, heart health, and blood sugar regulation.

Here are some ways to consume them:

1. Eat Fresh Bilberries

- Wash thoroughly and eat them raw as a snack.
- Add them to yogurt, smoothies, or oatmeal for a nutritious boost.

2. Make Bilberry Tea

- Boil 1 cup of water and add 1-2 teaspoons of dried bilberries.
- Let it steep for 10 minutes, strain, and enjoy.

3. Drink Bilberry Juice

- Blend fresh or frozen bilberries with water.
- Strain if necessary and drink pure or mix with other fruit juices.

Avaram Senna

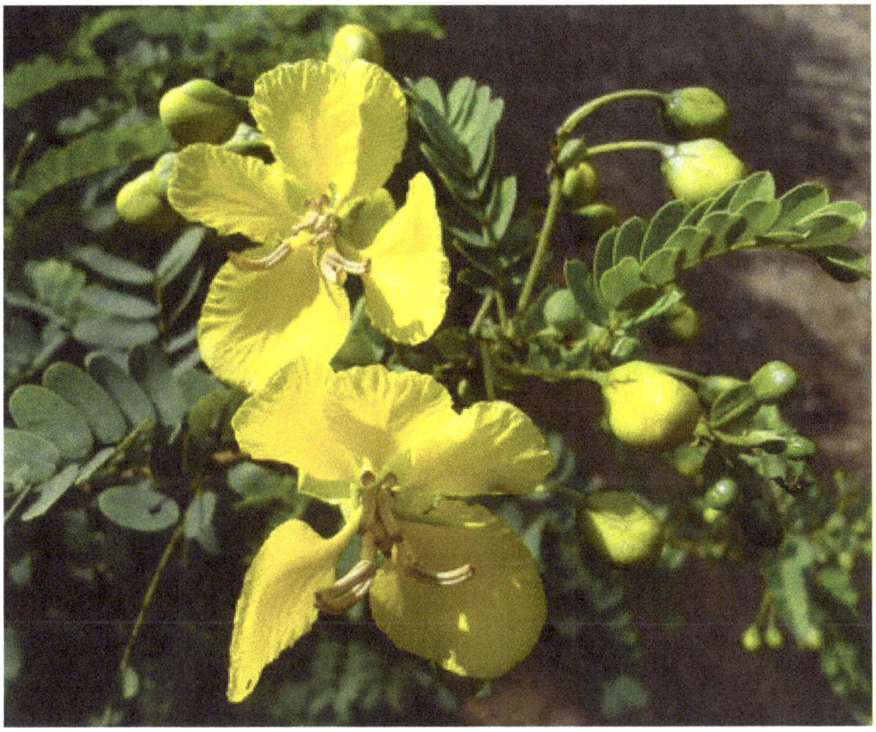

What is Avaram Senna?

Avaram Senna (Cassia auriculata) is a common tree in Asia, which has been widely used in Indian traditional medicine. The tree grows wildly and found abundantly near the river beds. Avaram Senna flower, which is called as Tanner's cassia is bright yellow in color. The dried flowers and buds have many therapeutic benefits. In Ayurveda, Avaram Senna flower is used for treating diabetes.

Scientific name: Senna auriculata

The root is used in decoctions against fevers, diabetes, diseases of urinary system and constipation. The leaves have laxative properties.

The dried flowers and flower buds are used as a substitute for tea in case of diabetes patients. The powdered seed is also applied to the eye, in case of chronic purulent conjunctivitis.

The wonder flower gives longevity to life. Avaram Senna flower is widely used as a home remedy for skin disorders and body odor. It is also used for the treatment of pain, fever, urinary tract disorders, rheumatism, conjunctivitis, ulcers and liver disease.

How to Consume Avaram Senna for Health Benefits

Avaram Senna (Senna auriculata), also known as Tanner's Cassia, is a powerful herb known for regulating blood sugar, improving skin health, and supporting digestion.

Here are the best ways to consume it:

1. Avaram Senna Tea

- Boil 1 teaspoon of dried Avaram Senna flowers or leaves in 1 cup of water.
- Let it steep for 5–10 minutes, strain, and drink.
- Consume once or twice daily for best results.

2. Avaram Senna Powder

- Mix ½ teaspoon of Avaram Senna powder in warm water or milk.
- Drink in the morning or before bed.
- Can also be added to smoothies for extra nutrition.

3. Avaram Senna Herbal Infusion

- Soak the flowers overnight in water and drink in the morning for cooling effects.
- Helps detox the body and improve skin complexion.

4. Avaram Senna in Face Packs (For External Use)

- Mix Avaram Senna powder with rose water and apply it as a face mask.
- Helps treat acne, blemishes, and oily skin.

Asafoetida

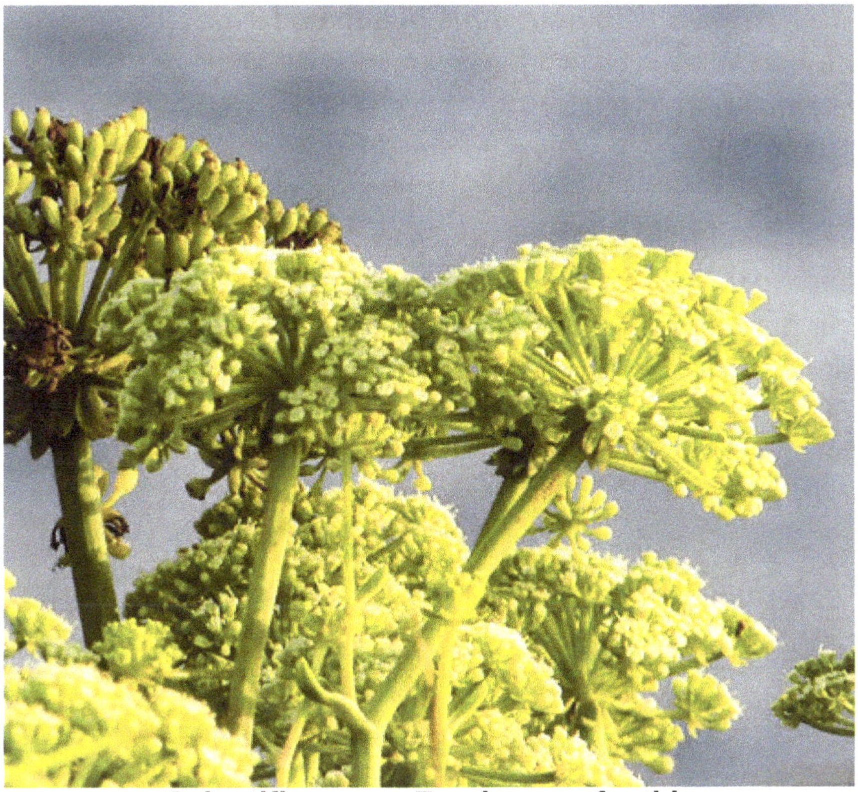

Scientific name: Ferula assa-foetida
Might be useful for IBS, high cholesterol, and breathing problems.

Asafoetida originates from India, where it's also called hing. Used for medicinal purposes and as a seasoning in many dishes, asafoetida has potential health benefits. Here's how to work it into your diet.

About Asafoetida

Ferula asafoetida comes from the fennel herb. Many parts of the plant are used in food and medicine. As a seasoning, it gives food an aromatic flavor. Gum resin is taken from the roots of the plant. It is used as a digestive aid, as a condiment, and in pickles.

It has a strong smell that is a mix of sulfur and onions. Adding a lot of this spice to a dish can overwhelm it. Once it cooks down, it takes more like a mild leek or garlic.

Health Benefits & How to Consume Asafoetida (Hing)

Asafoetida (Ferula assa-foetida), commonly known as Hing, is a powerful spice

with numerous health benefits:

1. **Aids Digestion** – Relieves bloating, gas, and constipation.
2. **Reduces Inflammation** – Helps with arthritis, asthma, and bronchitis.
3. **Regulates Blood Sugar** – May help control diabetes.
4. **Boosts Immunity** – Has antimicrobial and antiviral properties.
5. **Supports Heart Health** – Lowers blood pressure and improves circulation.
6. **Relieves Menstrual Cramps** – Acts as a natural pain reliever.
7. **Fights Respiratory Issues** – Clears mucus and relieves cough.
8. **Improves Mood** – Used in Ayurveda to reduce anxiety and depression.

How to Consume Asafoetida

1. Asafoetida Water (For Digestion & Gas Relief)

- Mix a pinch of Hing in a glass of warm water.
- Drink before meals to improve digestion.

2. Asafoetida Tea (For Cough & Cold)

- Boil 1 cup of water, add a pinch of Hing, honey, and ginger.
- Drink once or twice daily for respiratory relief.

3. Asafoetida Paste (For Menstrual Pain & Joint Pain)

- Mix Hing powder with warm water and apply to the lower abdomen for cramps.
- Apply a paste on swollen joints for pain relief.

4. Cooking with Asafoetida (Daily Use)

- Add a small pinch to soups, curries, and lentils for better digestion.
- Can be fried in ghee or oil to enhance flavor.

In herbal medicine, asafoetida is used to help treat:

- Asthma
- Bronchitis
- High blood pressure
- Nervous conditions
- Whooping cough

The gum resin has medicinal properties that may help with:

- Muscle spasms (antispasmodic)
- Intestinal gas (carminative)
- Cough (expectorant)
- Constipation (laxative)
- Calming (sedative)

Ashwagandha

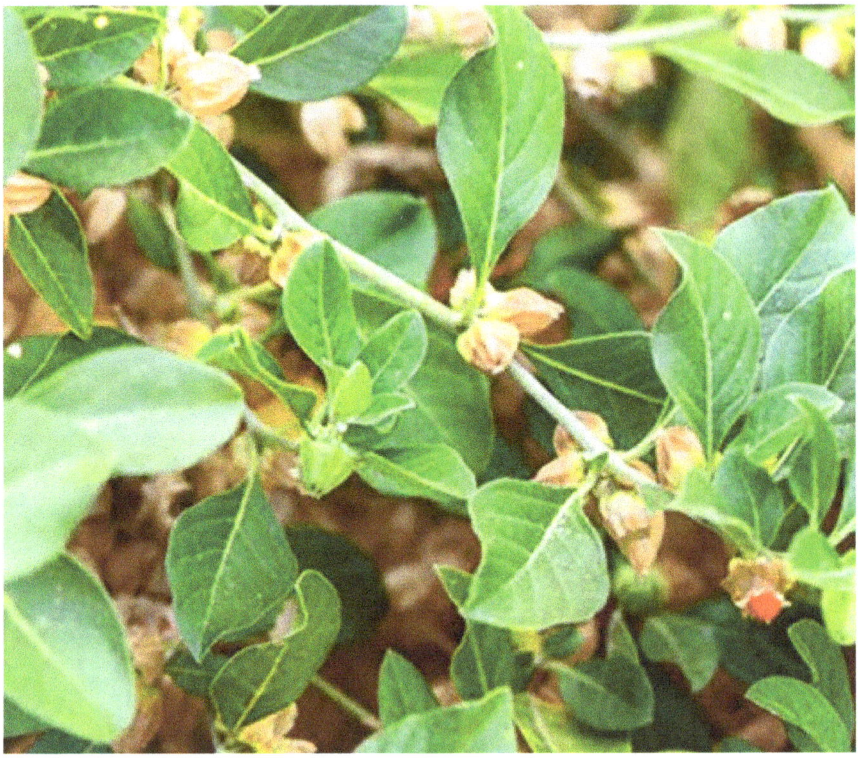

Ashwagandha is a popular adaptogenic herb offering numerous benefits for women's well-being. It can help promote a sense of calm while enhancing energy, helping you maintain balance with a clear mind and positive outlook.

Balance hormone levels

Ashwagandha's ability to balance hormones can be particularly beneficial for women's health, impacting aspects like the menstrual cycle, reproduction, and menopause.

2019 research suggests ashwagandha impacts the endocrine system, which governs mood, stress responses, and reproduction. This influence can help with hormonal imbalances, including anxiety, depression, and sleep issues.

Regulate menstrual cycle

Ashwagandha has a beneficial effect on key factors that influence your menstrual cycle, such as stress, inflammation, and hormonal fluctuations.
It helps regulate your cycle by balancing reproductive hormonesTrusted Source like serum follicle-stimulating hormone (FSH), luteinizing hormone (LH), and gonadotropin hormones. This balance may also be associated with a better balance of the stress hormone cortisol.

Conditions such as endometriosis, pelvic inflammatory disease (PID), and polycystic ovary syndrome (PCOS) often contribute to irregular menstrual cycles. Ashwagandha's phytoestrogens may help restore balance and aid in cycle regulation.

How to Consume Ashwagandha

Ashwagandha (Withania somnifera) is a powerful adaptogenic herb known for its stress-relieving, immune-boosting, and energy-enhancing properties. Here are the best ways to consume it:

1. Ashwagandha Powder (Churna)
(For Stress Relief & Energy)

- Mix ½ to 1 teaspoon of ashwagandha powder in warm milk or water.
- Add honey or a pinch of cinnamon for taste.
- Drink before bedtime for better sleep or in the morning for energy.

2. Ashwagandha Tea
(For Relaxation & Immunity)

- Boil 1 teaspoon of ashwagandha powder in 2 cups of water for 10 minutes.
- Strain and add honey or lemon for flavor.
- Drink once or twice daily.

Astragalus

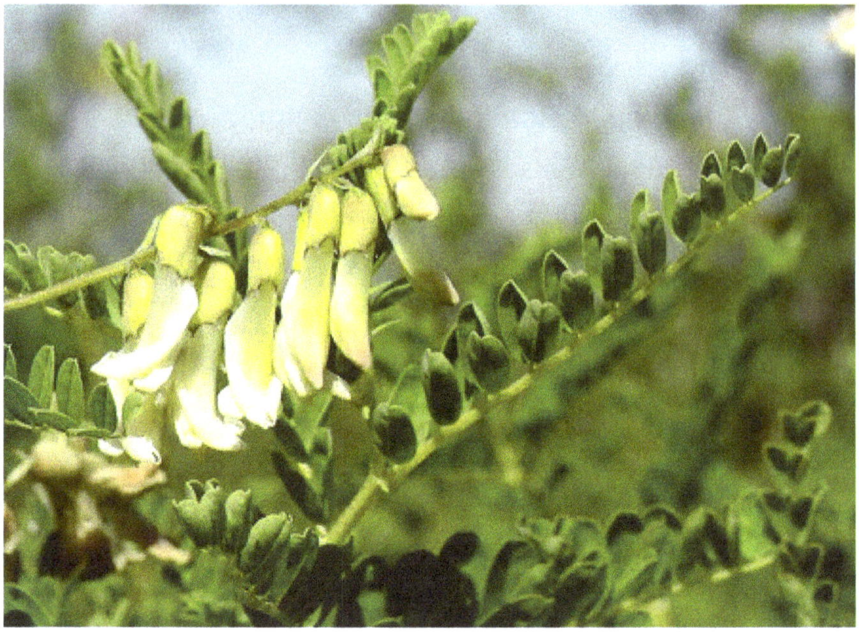

Scientific name: Astragalus propinquus
Long been used in traditional Chinese medicine to strengthen the immune system, and is used in modern China to treat hepatitis and as an adjunctive therapy in cancer.

What Is Astragalus Used For?

Astragalus is a natural dietary supplement that's used for various health conditions. For instance, it's used to treat the common cold, upper respiratory infections, fibromyalgia, and diabetes. Some proponents of astragalus use it for its possible heart benefits. They claim it may protect against heart disease. It's also used to help improve overall weakness.

Proponents also say astragalus stimulates the spleen, liver, lungs, circulatory, and urinary systems. It's also used to treat osteoarthritis, asthma, and nervous conditions as well as to lower blood sugar and blood pressure.

Astragalus is also known as Huang Qi, milkvetch, locoweed, and goat's-thorn. Only the root of the leafy astragalus is used, which contains the most active compounds and is usually harvested on plants around four years old. It can be dried and powdered, used raw and infused into teas, and turned into other supplements such as capsules and liquid extracts.

How to Consume Astragalus

Astragalus (Astragalus membranaceus) is an adaptogenic herb known for boosting immunity, reducing stress, and supporting heart health. It is commonly consumed in various forms, including teas, tinctures, and capsules.

1. Astragalus Tea (Best for Immunity & Energy)

Ingredients:

- 1-2 tablespoons of dried astragalus root (sliced or powdered)
- 2-3 cups of water
- Honey or lemon (optional)

How to Prepare:

- Boil water and add the astragalus root.
- Simmer for 15-30 minutes to extract the beneficial compounds.
- Strain and drink once or twice daily.
- Add honey or lemon for flavor.

2. Astragalus Capsules or Tablets (Best for Convenience)

Dosage:

- Take 500–1,500 mg daily (or as directed on the product label).
- Best taken with food for better absorption.

Barberry

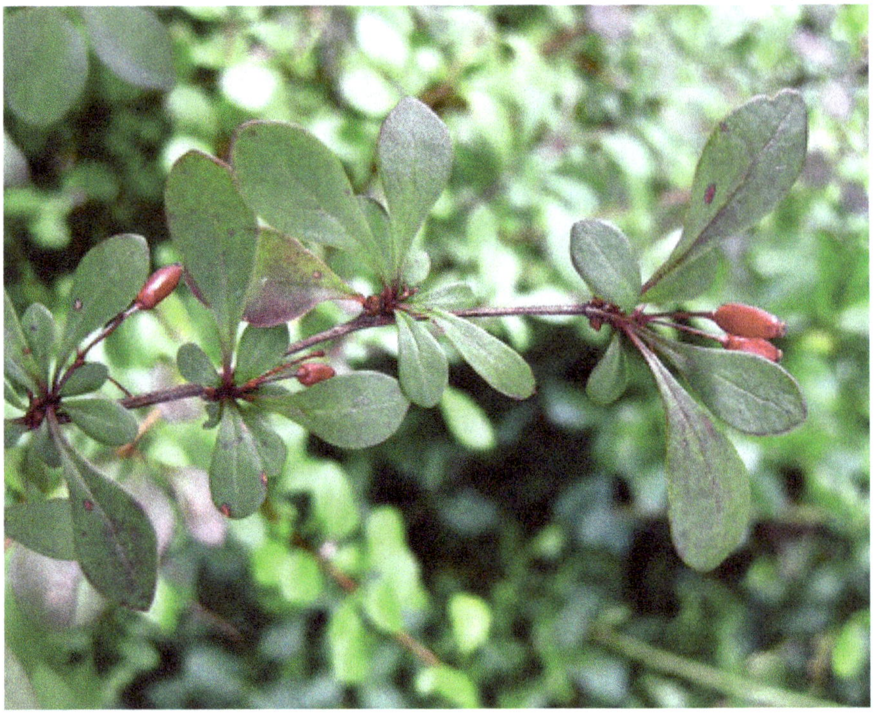

Scientific name: Berberis vulgaris

Long history of medicinal use, dating back to the Middle Ages particularly among Native Americans. Uses have included skin ailments, scurvy and gastro-intestinal ailments.

Health Benefits of Barberry:

Rich in Berberine

- Barberry contains berberine, a powerful plant compound known for its anti-inflammatory, antibacterial, and antioxidant properties.

Supports Digestive Health

- Traditionally used to ease digestive issues like indigestion, diarrhea, and upset stomach.
- Helps stimulate bile production and improve gut health.

Immune System Booster

- The antibacterial and antifungal properties help fight infections and strengthen the immune system.

Improves Heart Health

- May help reduce high blood pressure and cholesterol levels.
- Supports overall cardiovascular function.

Balances Blood Sugar

- Studies suggest barberry can help regulate blood sugar levels, making it beneficial for people with insulin resistance or type 2 diabetes.

Skin Health

- Used topically or taken internally to help clear acne, treat skin inflammation, and heal wounds.

Antioxidant Protection

- Protects cells from oxidative stress, helping reduce signs of aging and chronic inflammation.

How to Consume Barberry:

Barberry Tea

- Add 1–2 teaspoons of dried barberries to hot water and steep for 10 minutes. Drink 1–2 times a day.

Dried Barberries

- Can be sprinkled on salads, oatmeal, or used in cooking (popular in Persian rice dishes).
- Barberry Tincture or Extract
- Follow dosage instructions provided on the product label.

Barberry Capsules

Available in health food stores or online; always follow recommended dosages.

Caution:

Not recommended during pregnancy.
Always consult your healthcare provider before starting any herbal supplement, especially if you are on medication.

Bay Laurel

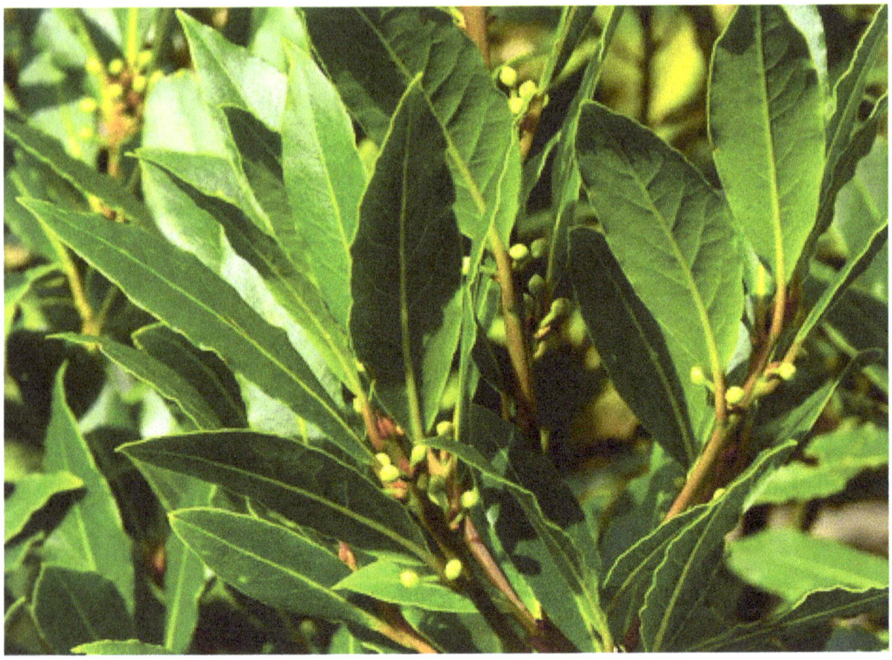

Scientific name: Laurus nobilis
Aqueous extracts of bay laurel can be used as astringents and even as a reasonable salve for open wounds.
In massage therapy, the essential oil of bay laurel is reputed to alleviate arthritis and rheumatism, while in aromatherapy it is used to treat earaches and high blood pressure.

Bay leaf (also known as laurel) is a spice commonly used to flavor soups and meat dishes for its light, herbal flavor. It is sometimes sold in stores in a powder or as a fresh leaf, but it is most often found as a dry, whole leaf. You add the leaf during cooking and take it out before serving, since it's tough to chew and digest.

Some people believe that bay leaves are poisonous, but that's not true.
There are many species in the bay leaf family, but all share a similar taste and nutrition profile. Varieties of the bay leaf can be grown everywhere from the Caribbean to India, and it is found in the spice aisles of grocery stores around the world.

Bay Leaf Benefits

It adds minimal calories to your food while boosting the amount of fiber, vitamins, minerals, and antioxidants.

Some notable health benefits of bay leaf include:
Immune system health. Bay leaf is a good source of vitamin A, vitamin B6, and vitamin C. These vitamins are all known to support a healthy immune system.

How to Consume Bay Leaf Safely and Effectively:

1. Bay Leaf Tea

- Add 2–3 dried bay leaves to a cup of boiling water.
- Let it steep for 5–10 minutes, remove the leaves, and sip warm.
- Can be consumed 1–2 times daily for relaxation, digestive support, or to reduce inflammation.

2. Cooking with Bay Leaves

- Add 1–2 dried bay leaves to soups, stews, sauces, rice, or meat dishes while cooking.
- Remove the bay leaves before serving (they are not meant to be eaten whole).

3. Bay Leaf Infused Water

- Add 3–4 bay leaves to a jug of water and let it sit overnight.
- Drink throughout the day for gentle detox and digestive aid

4. Bay Leaf Essential Oil (External Use Only)

- Can be diluted with a carrier oil and used for massages to ease muscle pain and improve circulation.

Chamomile

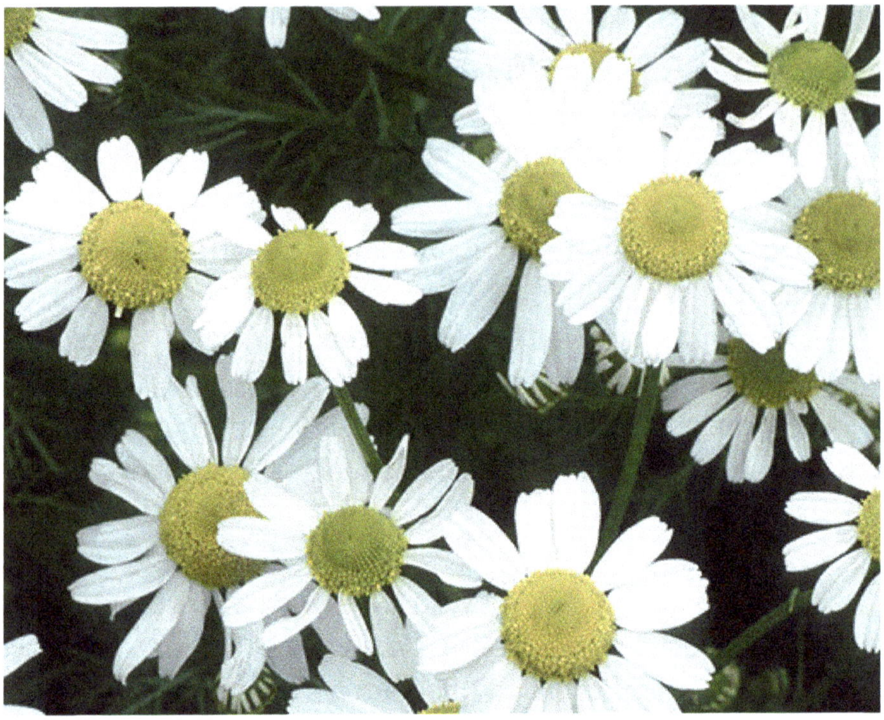

Chamomile tea is a natural remedy for a wide range of health issues. The nutrients it contains may help manage diabetes, menstrual pain, and sleep problems, among others.

Chamomile is a herb that belongs to the Asteraceae family. There are two common varieties of chamomile that people often use for tea: German (Chamomilla recutita) and Roman (Chamaemelum nobile). The chamomile plant produces small flowers similar to daisies, that people can dry and steep in water to make tea.

Chamomile Tea Health Benefits:

Promotes Better Sleep

- Chamomile contains apigenin, a natural compound that helps calm the nervous system and improves sleep quality.

- Drinking a warm cup before bedtime can help fight insomnia and restlessness.

- Reduces Stress and Anxiety Chamomile is known for its relaxing properties and can ease symptoms of anxiety and tension.

Supports Digestive Health

- Helps relieve bloating, indigestion, nausea, and gas.
- Can soothe an upset stomach and reduce cramps.

Anti-Inflammatory Properties

- Chamomile can reduce inflammation in the body and may help ease joint pain and muscle soreness.

Boosts Immune System

- Regular consumption may help strengthen immunity and protect against common colds and infections.

Helps Menstrual Cramps

- Chamomile tea can ease period pain by relaxing uterine muscles and reducing tension.

Improves Skin Health

- The antioxidants in chamomile promote healthy skin and can reduce acne, irritation, and redness.

How to Prepare Chamomile Tea:

- Add 1–2 teaspoons of dried chamomile flowers or 1 tea bag to a cup of boiling water.Steep for 5–10 minutes.

- Sweeten with honey if desired.
- Drink 1–2 cups per day for relaxation and wellness benefits.

Caution:

Avoid excessive use if allergic to ragweed or related plants.
Consult your doctor if you're pregnant, breastfeeding, or on blood thinners.

Tamarind

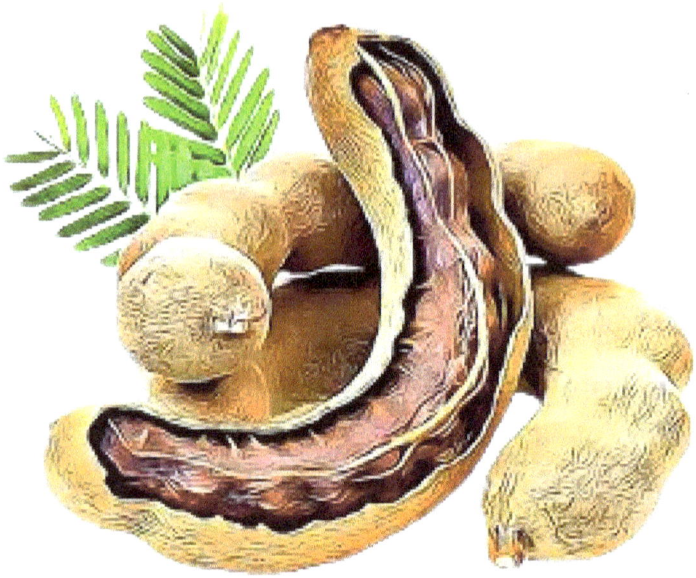

Health Benefits of Tamarind

The tamarind tree is much prized in many parts of the world for its beauty and its fruit. Tamarinds are leguminous trees because they produce fruit in the form of a bean-like pod. This bean contains a sour pulp that becomes very sweet as it ripens. People eat the fruit raw and also use its pulp in cooking.

The leaves, beans, bark, and wood of the tamarind tree have a wide variety of uses. Tamarind is an ingredient in Worcestershire sauce and is used in many dishes in Asia, South and Central America, Africa, and the Caribbean. It appears in many chutneys, sauces, candies, and drinks.

Health Benefits

People use tamarind in traditional medicine, but its therapeutic uses need more exploration. Tamarind pulp contains a variety of nutrients that can boost your health.

Tissue Health

Amino acids, the building blocks of protein, are necessary for the body to grow and repair tissues. Some amino acids are essential, meaning that the body can't synthesize them, so people must get them from food. Tamarind contains significant amounts of all the essential amino acids except tryptophan.

Tamarind Leaf Benefits:

- Anti-inflammatory Properties
- Tamarind leaves are known to help reduce swelling, joint pain, and muscle aches.
- Often used in traditional remedies for arthritis and rheumatism.

Boosts Immunity

- Rich in antioxidants and vitamin C, tamarind leaves help strengthen the immune system and protect against infections.

Improves Digestion

- Tamarind leaves can help relieve indigestion, stomach cramps, and diarrhea.
- They promote healthy bowel movements and cleanse the digestive tract.

Helps Manage Fever

- Tamarind leaf decoctions are traditionally used to reduce fever and cool the body.

Promotes Skin Health

- The antibacterial properties can help treat skin infections, rashes, and wounds when applied as a paste.

Liver Detoxification

- Consuming tamarind leaf tea or juice helps flush toxins from the liver and supports liver health.

Supports Respiratory Health

- Tamarind leaves are used in remedies for coughs, asthma, and bronchitis, helping clear mucus and ease breathing

How to Consume Tamarind Leaves:

Tamarind Leaf Tea:

- Boil a handful of fresh or dried tamarind leaves in water for 10 minutes.
- Strain and drink 1–2 cups daily for detox and immune support.

Bone Health

People who get enough magnesium in their diets have better bone density than those who are deficient. Many people, especially teens and those over 70, do not get adequate magnesium. Tamarind is a rich source of magnesium. It also contains more calcium than many plant foods.

The combination of these two minerals, plus weight-bearing exercise, could help prevent osteoporosis and bone fractures. The body requires vitamin D to use calcium. Tamarind is not a significant source of vitamin D, so you will need to get it from other sources.

Nutrition

Tamarind is very rich in nutrients, providing at least 10% of:

- Vitamin B1 (Thiamine)
- Vitamin B3 (Niacin)
- Potassium
- Magnesium
- Phosphorus
- Iron

Lemon Balm

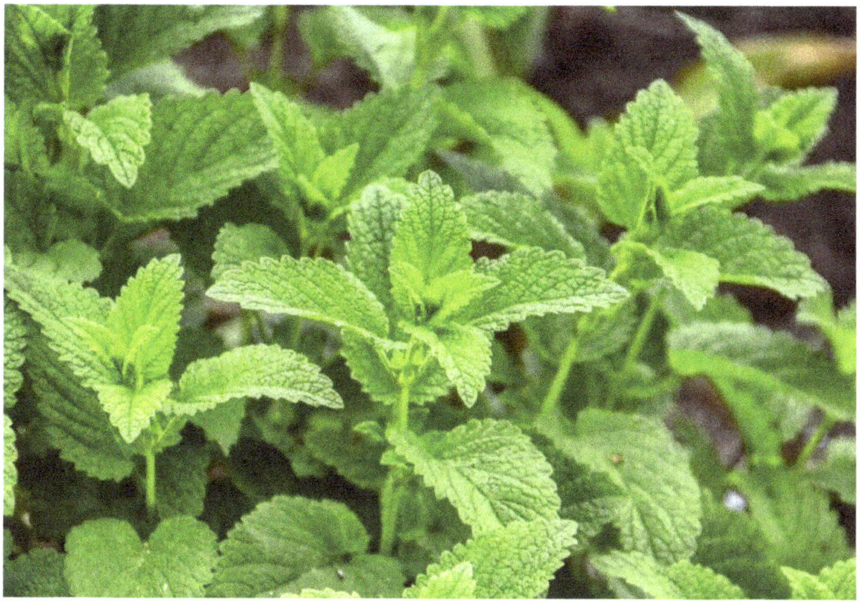

What Is Lemon Balm?
Lemon balm, known as a calming herb, helps everything from anxiety to indigestion. It's a perennial member of the mint family, and its leaves have a light lemon fragrance.

Lemon balm is known by many other names, such as bee balm, cure-all, dropsy plant, honey plant, garden balm, heart's delight, sweet balm, and sweet Mary.
Native to southern Europe, the Mediterranean, and Central Asia, the lemon balm plant can be found in many parts of the world. Its small white flowers attract bees and other pollinators, while its lemony scent repels mosquitoes.

Lemon balm has been used as medicine for over a thousand years. It's believed to help with various disorders.

Lemon Balm Benefits
Studies have shown that the herb is a potential treatment for many issues, from anxiety to menstrual symptoms.
Lemon balm may provide the following health benefits:
Reducing anxiety
If you need to relieve stress, lemon balm can help lower anxiety and nervousness.

Some research has shown that lemon balm extract can improve one's mood and attention. A study found that chemicals called terpenes found in lemon balm can help calm agitation in people with severe dementia by reactivating brain circuits.

Treating insomnia

- Research has shown that when combined with herbs like valerian, lemon balm helps improve sleep. Also, drinking lemon balm tea can help with insomnia.

Easing digestive problems

- Compounds in lemon balm may relieve gastrointestinal problems such as bloating and indigestion.

Healing cold sores

- Lemon balm ointments have been found to help heal cold sores caused by the herpes simplex virus (HSV).

Easing menstrual pain

- The compound rosmarinic acid in lemon balm may help minimize the severity of menstrual symptoms like cramps and fatigue.

Improving memory

- Lemon balm may help with brain functions like memory, learning, focus, and mood.

Boosting cardiovascular health

- Research suggests that lemon balm may promote heart health. A 2021 review highlighted that lemon balm may help with cardiovascular health by improving low or high blood pressure and high heart rate.

Echinacea

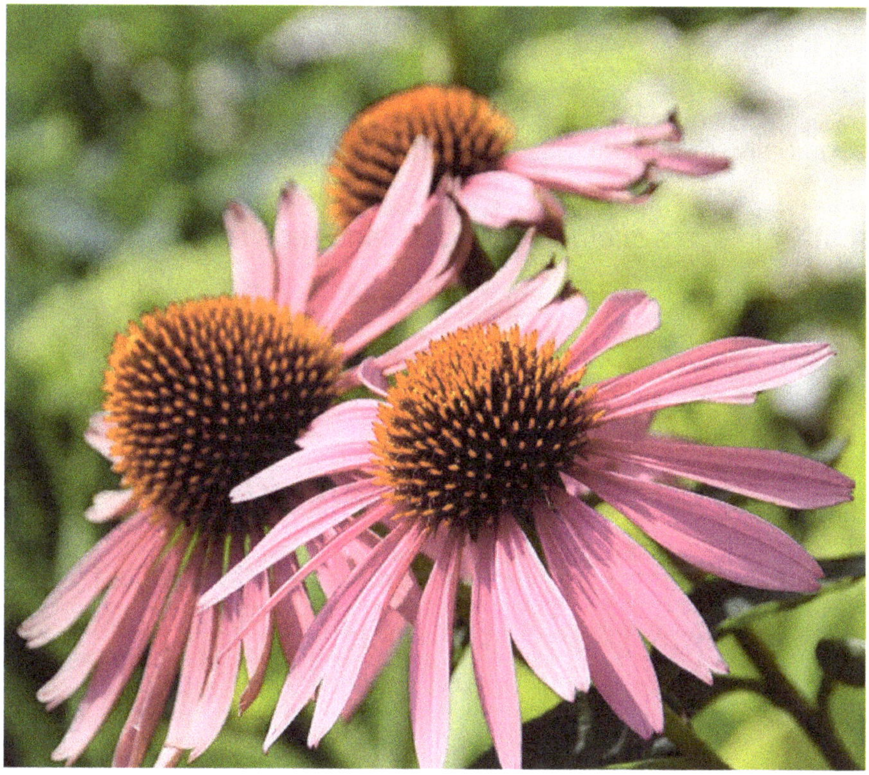

Echinacea is one of the most popular herbs in America today. Echinacea is a Native American medicinal plant named for the prickly scales in its large conical seed head, which resembles the spines of an angry hedgehog (echinos is Greek for hedgehog).

Archaeologists have found evidence that Native Americans may have used echinacea for more than 400 years to treat infections and wounds, and as a general "cure-all." Throughout history people have used echinacea to treat scarlet fever, syphilis, malaria, blood poisoning, and diphtheria. Although this herb was popular during the 18th and 19th centuries, its use began to decline in the United States after the introduction of antibiotics.

Echinacea preparations became increasingly popular in Germany throughout the 20th century. In fact, most of the scientific research on echinacea has been conducted in Germany.

Today, people use echinacea to shorten the duration of the common cold and flu, and reduce symptoms, such as sore throat (pharyngitis), cough, and fever. Many herbalists also recommend echinacea to help boost the immune system and help the body fight infections.

How to Consume Echinacea:

Method:

- Steep 1–2 teaspoons of dried Echinacea root, leaves, or flowers in hot water for 10–15 minutes.
- Drink 1–3 cups daily, especially at the onset of cold or flu symptoms.
- Benefit:
- Helps boost the immune system, fights colds, and reduces inflammation.

Echinacea Tincture

Method:

- Take 1–2 droppers (about 20–40 drops) in water or juice, 2–3 times per day.
- Benefit:
- Quick-acting and concentrated for immune support and faster symptom relief.

Mint

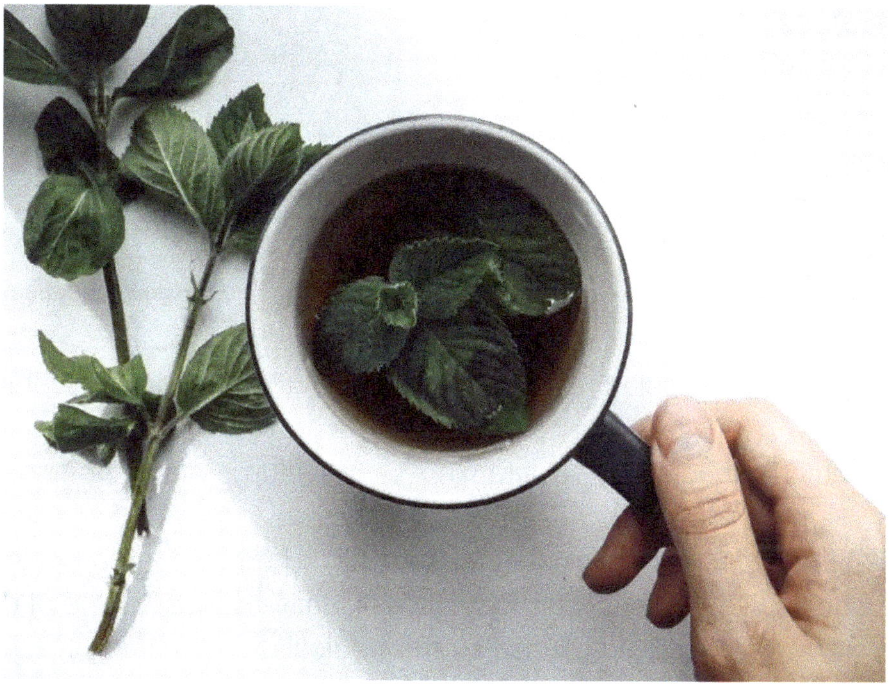

Mint is a fragrant and delicious plant that is an ingredient in many foods and beverages. It also has health benefits that may include relieving indigestion, improving brain function, and masking bad breath.

Mint is the name for over a dozen plant species, including peppermint and spearmint, that belong to the genus Mentha.
These plants are particularly known for the cooling sensation they impart. They can be added to foods in both fresh and dried forms.

Mint is a popular ingredient in several foods and beverages, ranging from teas and alcoholic drinks to sauces, salads and desserts.

While eating the plant offers some health benefits, research shows that several of mint's health benefits come from applying it to the skin, inhaling its aroma or taking it as a capsule.

While not typically consumed in large quantities, mint does contain a fair amount of nutrients.

In fact, just 2 tablespoons (11.4 grams) of spearmint contains:

- Calories: 5
- Fiber: 0.8 grams
- Vitamin A: 3% of the Daily Value
- Iron: 8% of the DV
- Manganese: 6% of the DV
- Folate: 3% of the DV

Because of its dynamic flavor, mint is often added to recipes in small amounts, so consuming even 2 tablespoons may be difficult. However, it's possible you may come close to this amount in some salad recipes that include mint among the other ingredients.

Mint is a particularly good source of vitamin A, a fat-soluble vitamin that is critical for eye health and night vision.
It is also a potent source of antioxidants, especially when compared to other herbs and spices. Antioxidants help protect your body from oxidative stress, a type of damage to cells caused by free radicals.

Making mint tea is super simple and refreshing! You can use either fresh or dried mint leaves, depending on what you have. Here's how to make it both ways:

Ingredients:

- A handful of fresh mint leaves (10–15 leaves)
- 2 cups of water
- Optional: honey, lemon, or ginger

Instructions:

1. Rinse the mint leaves gently to remove any dirt.
2. Boil the water in a pot or kettle.
3. Once it boils, remove from heat and add the mint leaves.
4. Cover and steep for 5–10 minutes (longer = stronger flavor).
5. Strain into a cup, sweeten if desired, and enjoy!

Banana Peel

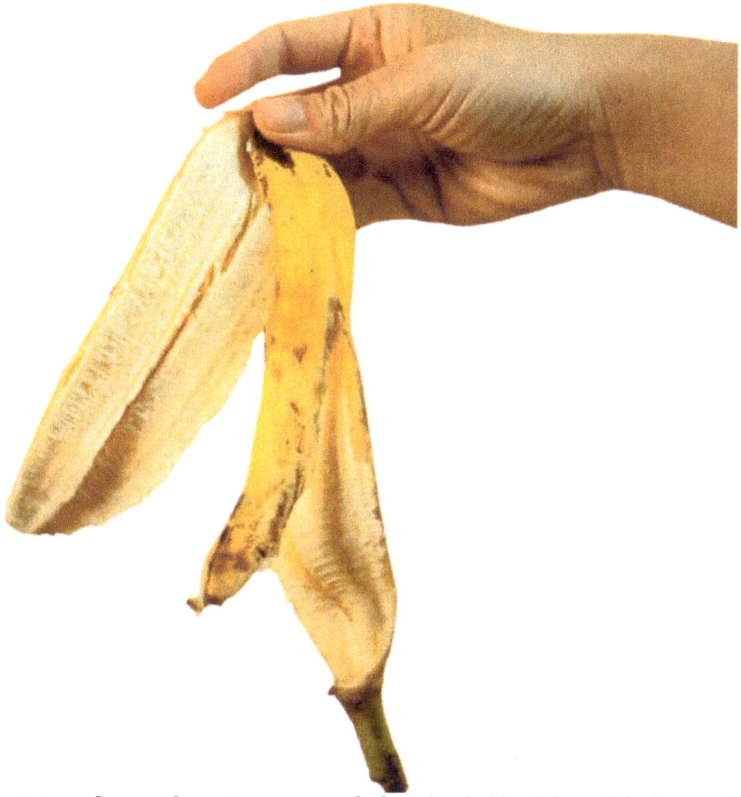

Banana peels aren't just trash — they're surprisingly full of health benefits! Here's what they can do:

Digestive Health

- Fiber-rich banana peels can help regulate the digestive system, easing both constipation and diarrhea. This can be a particularly important benefit of banana peels for people with Crohn's disease or irritable bowel syndrome.

Better Eyesight

- Vitamin A can help keep your eyes strong and healthy. This vitamin is abundant in both bananas and banana peels.

May Lower Cancer Risk

- Banana peels are packed with polyphenols, carotenoids, and other antioxidants that fight cancer-causing free radicals in your body. Eating more banana peels, especially green, unripe peels, can increase your antioxidant levels and help reduce your risk of cancer.

Health Benefits

Both bananas and banana peels may offer different health benefits depending on their level of ripeness. Underripe, green bananas may be more effective in treating digestive issues, while riper, blackened bananas have been shown to help white blood cells fight off disease and infection.

Depression Relief

The high levels of tryptophan in bananas, combined with the B6 in banana peels, can help relieve some symptoms of depression and other mood disorders. Tryptophan turns into serotonin as it breaks down, which can improve your mood. Vitamin B6 can help improve sleep, which has a positive impact on mood over time.

How to Consume Banana Peel

Banana peels are rich in fiber, antioxidants, and essential nutrients like potassium, magnesium, and vitamin B6. They can be eaten in various ways to boost digestion, heart health, and mood.

Banana Peel Tea (For Relaxation & Sleep Aid)

Ingredients:

- 1 ripe banana peel (organic, washed)
- 2 cups of water
- Honey or cinnamon (optional)

How to Prepare:

- Cut the banana peel into small pieces.
- Boil in 2 cups of water for 10-15 minutes.
- Strain and enjoy with honey or cinnamon.
- Drink before bedtime for relaxation.

Pumpkin Seeds

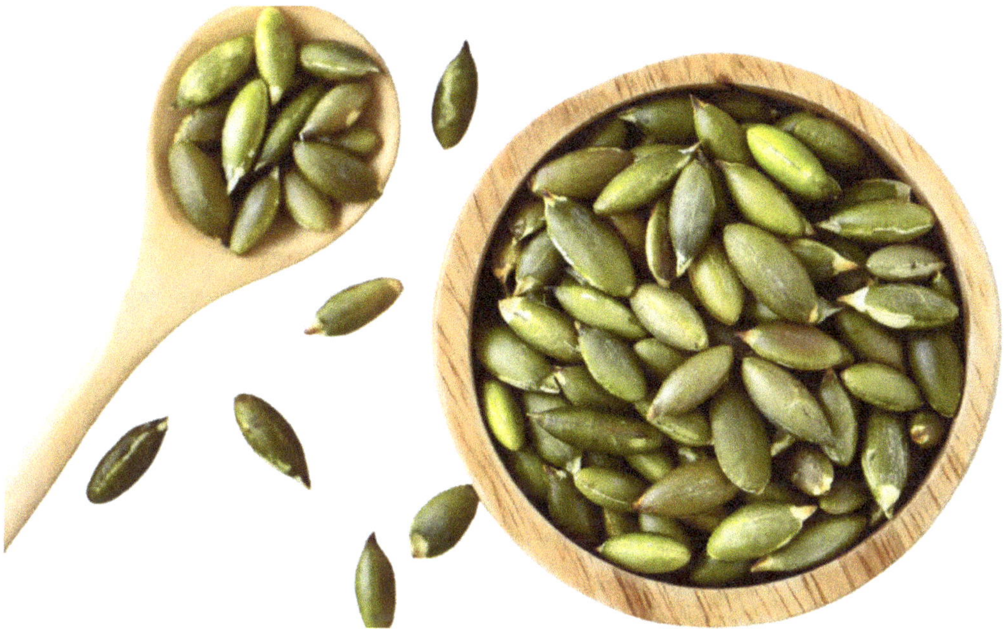

Pumpkin seeds (aka pepitas) are tiny powerhouses packed with nutrients and health benefits. Here's why they deserve a spot in your diet:

Health Benefits of Pumpkin Seeds

Pumpkin seeds are a rich source of protein, unsaturated fatty acids, vitamins, and minerals that may reduce your risk of getting chronic diseases, such as cancer.
Some potential health benefits include:

Anti-inflammatory effects

Pumpkin seeds are rich in many antioxidants, which protect your cells from disease-causing damage and reduce inflammation in your body. When they have their hulls, they're also a great source of dietary fiber, which can boost this effect. Studies show that anti-inflammatory foods can help you prevent chronic diseases, such as type 2 diabetes and heart disease.

Improved prostate health

Several studies have shown that pumpkin seeds may help ease the symptoms of benign prostatic hyperplasia (BPH). BPH is a condition where your prostate gland is swollen. This can cause it to press against your urethra and irritate your bladder. People with BPH may feel as if they have to pee all the time or they may be unable to completely empty their bladder.

But medicines that treat BPH, such as alpha-blockers and 5-alpha-reductase inhibitors (5ARIs), can have side effects like sexual function disorders that may not go away even if you stop taking the medicine.

How to Consume Pumpkin Seeds:

1. Raw Pumpkin Seeds

- Eat them as a healthy snack by the handful.
- Add to salads, yogurt, or oatmeal for extra crunch and nutrients.

2. Roasted Pumpkin Seeds

Method:

- Toss raw seeds with olive oil and a pinch of salt or your favorite spices.
- Bake at 300°F (150°C) for 20–30 minutes, stirring occasionally until golden.
- Delicious as a snack or topping for soups and salads.

3. Pumpkin Seed Butter

- Spread on toast, crackers, or add to smoothies for a creamy, nutty flavor.
- You can buy it or make your own by blending roasted seeds until smooth.

4. Pumpkin Seed Powder

- Add 1–2 tablespoons to smoothies, shakes, or baking recipes for a protein and magnesium boost.

5. Pumpkin Seed Oil

- Use as a salad dressing drizzle or over roasted vegetables (do not cook at high heat).

Health Benefits of Pumpkin Seeds:

- Rich in magnesium, zinc, and antioxidants.
- Supports heart health, prostate health, and immune function.
- Promotes better sleep (high in tryptophan).
- Great for skin and hair health.

Sorrel

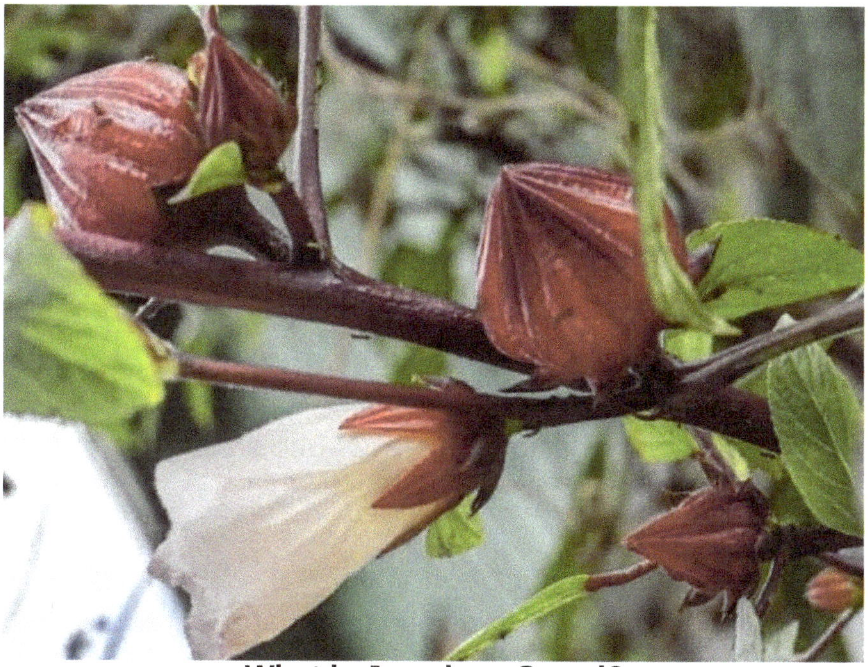

What is Jamaican Sorrel?

I have to make clear what Jamaican sorrel is not before saying what it is, because there is a lot of confusion and it often gets mixed up with other plants. Don't confuse Rumex acetosa or Rumex acetosella, which are also called sorrel, with Jamaican sorrel. These are leafy green herbs that resemble spinach and used in salad and other cuisines.

Some people also think that hibiscus is Jamaican sorrel. Although Jamaican sorrel is apart of the hibiscus family it should not be mistaken for hibiscus.
Jamaican sorrel and other plants from the hibiscus family are sorted after because of the tremendous amount of health benefits that comes with consuming the plant.

Below are 9 health benefits that are known to drinking Jamaican sorrel drink.

1. Weight loss

- Studies have suggested that there is an acid in sorrel that helps with weight loss.

- This acid discharge more amylase (an enzyme that helps you digest food) into the digestive system, which breaks down excess starch and sugar (calories) molecules in the body.

- A regular intake of sorrel will improve weight gain.

2. Anti- cancer

- The anthocyanin and antioxidant properties found in sorrel are known to prevent the development of cancer cells in the body.

3. Anti – inflammatory

- The anti-inflammatory properties found in sorrel helps to neutralise the free radicals in our bodies that cause inflammatory conditions such as rheumatoid arthritis, eczema, stomach, and even cancer.

4. Lower blood pressure

- Sorrel has antihypertensive properties that help to lower blood pressure. A research done at a university in Boston found that persons who drink a cup of sorrel daily saw a significant reduction in their blood pressure level in 30 days.

5. Good Vision

- There is a high level of vitamin A that contributes to good vision.

6. Prevent heart disease

- Sorrel helps to keep the heart healthy and prevents the development of the cardiovascular disease. The powerful antioxidant properties in the sorrel reduce the bad cholesterols in the body that develop into heart disease.

7. Prevent flu and cold

- The sorrel is an ancient African remedy for cold and flu. The high vitamin C in sorrel can help to boost the immune system and help prevent the cold or flu.

8. Relief fever

- Because of the ability to cool the body down, sorrel can also reduce the effect of

9. Reduce menstrual cramps

- Drinking sorrel tea a few days before your period starts can ease menstruation cramps.

Sorrel is a tangy, vibrant herb and flower used in both culinary and herbal traditions—especially popular in the Caribbean (like the deep red hibiscus "sorrel drink") and in European cooking (where green sorrel leaves are used in soups and salads). Here's how you can consume it in different ways:

Hibiscus Sorrel (Jamaican Style)

Ingredients:

- 1–2 cups dried sorrel (hibiscus petals)
- 5–6 cups water
- 1–2 inches fresh ginger, sliced
- 5–10 whole cloves
- Sugar or honey (to taste)
- Optional: orange peel, cinnamon stick, pimento seeds, or a splash of rum

Instructions:

1. Boil water with ginger, cloves, and spices.
2. Add dried sorrel to the pot, stir, and let steep for several hours (overnight is best).
3. Strain the liquid through a fine sieve or cheesecloth.
4. Sweeten with sugar or honey.
5. Chill and serve over ice. Add rum for a festive twist!

Dog Blood

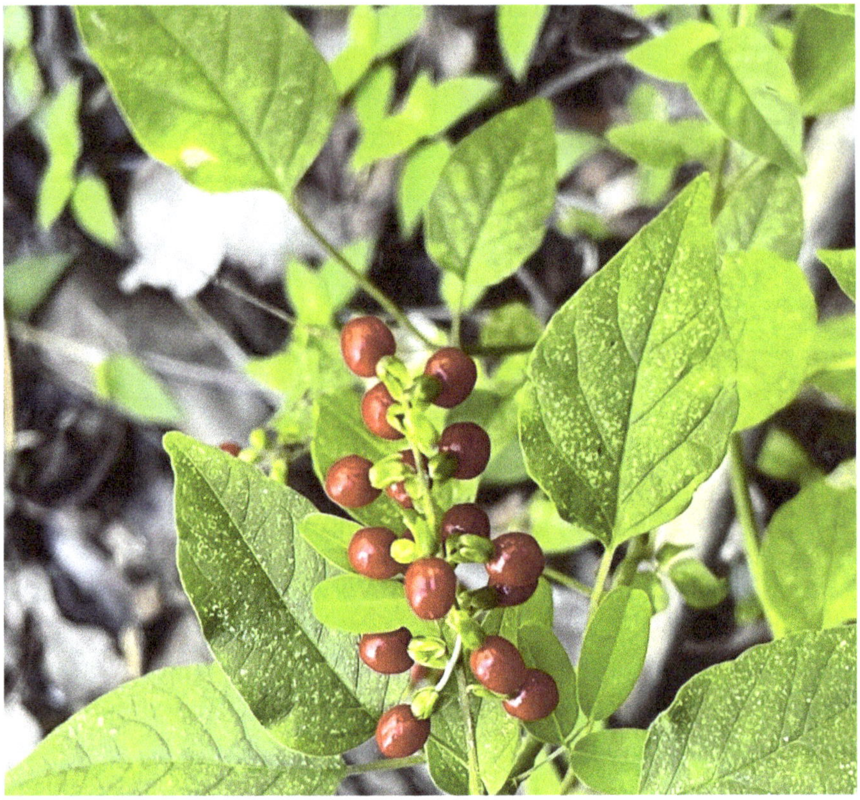

The dream of giving birth, raising children and truly tapping into the nurturing side, for some women, doesn't go much further than a reverie.

For those women, despite the latest medical interventions, money spent on fertility kits, and numerous pieces of advice from medical professionals, the desire to bring forth a child has never been realised.

But herbalists have touted the dog blood plant (Rivina Humilis), also called blood berry, rouge plant, baby pepper and fertility bush, as one natural solution to fertility issues.

According to nutritionist Donovan Grant, the plant, which features red berries, is said to clean the Fallopian tubes due to its anti-inflammatory properties, because inflammation in the tubes is a major cause of infertility.

Grant added that consuming dog blood bush is usually done by taking a cup of the boiled bush tea each day for a month.
The herbal concoction can also be used to treat period cramps.

Grant said in this case, one would need to drink a cup per day, starting three days before the period is due, and this may be combined with the Vervain bush in this regard.

Manchester-based herbalist Kneale Smith, however, said the bush has to be combined with two other herbs called clary (Wild Clary) and 'inflammation weed' after a proper body cleanse is done, for it to work.

"Our bodies are our temples and we have to watch what we put in it. Also, we must cleanse our bodies every quarter or at least three times per year," he said.

To make Dog Blood Bush tea, add 1 teaspoon of the dried herb to one cup of hot water, cover, and let it steep for 5-10 minutes before straining and enjoying.
Here's a more detailed breakdown:

1. Gather your ingredients: You'll need 1 teaspoon of dried Dog Blood Bush (Rivina humilis) herb and 1 cup of hot water.
2. Heat your water: Bring the water to a boil, then let it cool slightly before adding the herb.
3. Steep the herb: Place the 1 teaspoon of Dog Blood Bush herb in a cup or teapot.
4. Pour hot water: Pour the hot water over the herb, cover the cup, and let it steep for 5-10 minutes.
5. Strain the tea: After steeping, strain the tea to remove the herb leaves.
6. Enjoy: You can drink the tea warm or let it cool to your preference.

Cilantro

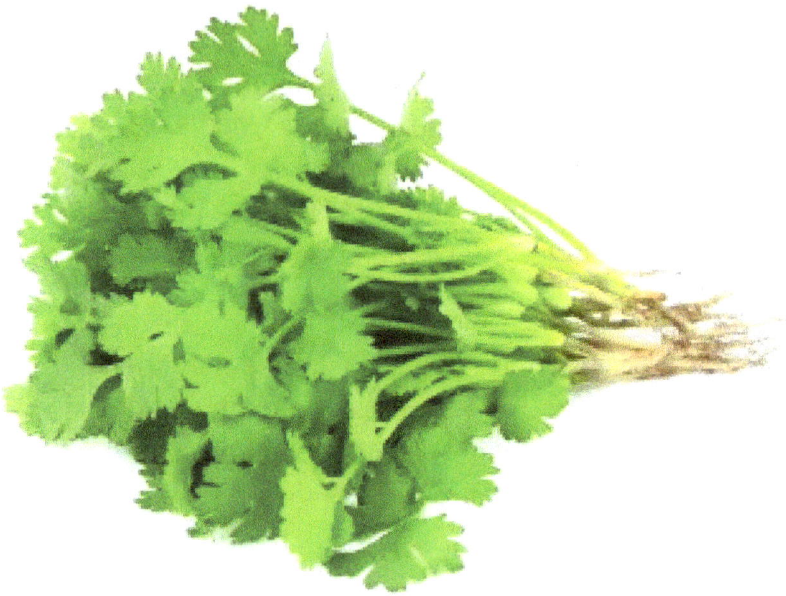

Cilantro leaves are rich in folate important for the formation of DNA and RNA, protein metabolism and regulating homocysteine levels. Maintaining low homocysteine levels may prevent damage to artery walls and risk of heart attack and stroke. Vitamin K is important for blood clotting and heart and bone health.

Health Benefits

Like many culinary herbs, cilantro has been used medicinally since ancient times. Modern research methods are finding support for some of the health claims attributed to this plant. Some health benefits of cilantro may include:

Brain Health

Although further research is still needed, several studies have connected eating cilantro with reduced symptoms of cognitive diseases like Alzheimer's and Parkinson's disease.

Blood Sugar Management

Cilantro is so well-known for its ability to lower blood sugar that people with low blood sugar or those taking diabetes medications are warned to be careful with the herb.
In animal studies, coriander seeds reduced blood sugar by stimulating an enzyme that removes sugar from the blood.

Prevent Foodborne Illnesses

The cilantro plant contains dodecenal, an antimicrobial compound that may help protect your body against infections and illnesses caused by tainted food. The compound is effective against Salmonella, a microbe that can cause life-threatening food poisoning.

Another study found that compounds in cilantro are effective against several bacteria, including those that cause foodborne illnesses and hospital-acquired infections.

How to Consume Cilantro (Coriander Leaves)

1. Fresh in Salads

- Chop fresh cilantro leaves and add to salads for a fresh, zesty flavor.

2. As a Garnish

- Sprinkle over soups, stews, tacos, curries, and rice dishes just before serving for a burst of freshness.

3. In Smoothies or Juices

- Blend a handful of cilantro with fruits, greens, and lemon juice for a detoxifying smoothie.

Celery

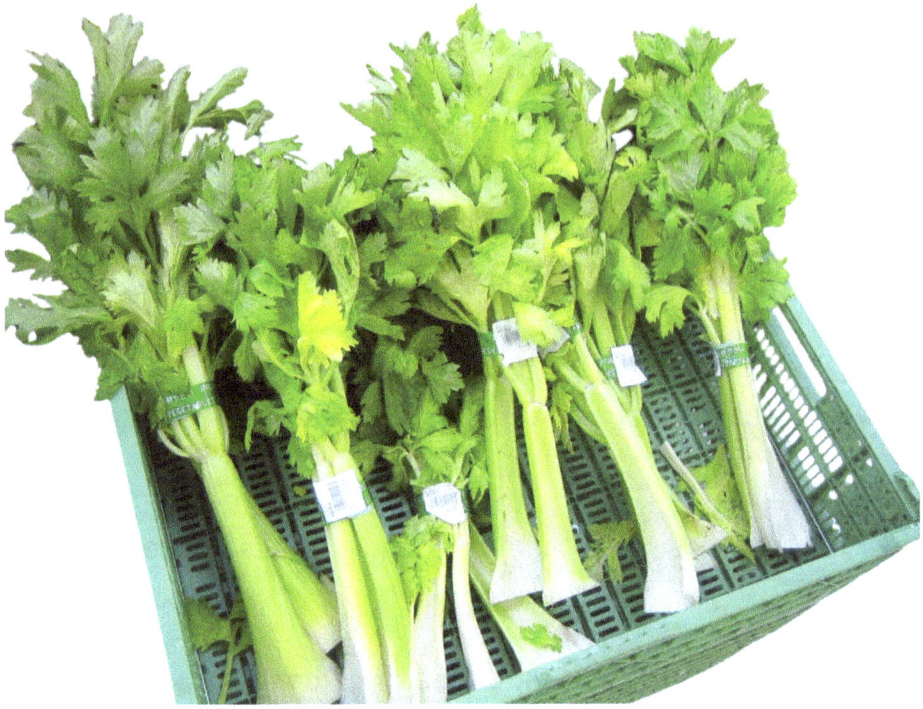

Celery is high in fiber and nutrients and low in calories. It's full of potassium , vitamins, and antioxidants. Celery is 95% water. It's a great snack if you're trying to lose weight or for regular bowel movements.

Cancer prevention

The antioxidants in celery include well-known varieties such as flavonoids and vitamin C, as well as lunularin and bergapten. They help cancel out natural chemicals in your body called free radicals that can harm cells and lead to cancer and other diseases.

Blood pressure management

Celery is rich in a plant compound called phthalide. This phytochemical relaxes your artery walls to help blood flow and to lower your blood pressure.

Alzheimer's disease prevention and treatment

Research in mice suggests that a compound called DL-3-n-butylphthalide made from seeds in the flowers of the celery plant improves learning, thinking, and memory. This seed extract may possibly treat and prevent Alzheimer's, but more studies are needed to confirm these benefits in the human population.

Celery is a powerhouse when it comes to health benefits, and you can consume it in several simple ways depending on what you're aiming for—whether it's detox, digestion, inflammation reduction, or general wellness.

1. Celery Juice (Popular for Detox & Digestion)

- How: Blend 4–6 stalks of celery with a little water, strain (optional), and drink on an empty stomach in the morning.
- Tip: You can add a bit of cucumber or apple for taste, but purists recommend it straight for the best results.

2. Raw Celery (Snacking & Salads)

- How: Eat raw celery sticks as a snack—great with hummus, peanut butter, or yogurt-based dips.
- Chop it into salads for a crunchy, hydrating element.

3. Cooked Celery (Soups, Stir-fries, Stews)

- How: Add chopped celery to your soups, stews, or stir-fries.
- Why: Cooking makes it easier to digest, though it slightly reduces the vitamin content.

4. Celery Seeds (For Blood Pressure & Inflammation)

- How: Use celery seed as a spice in cooking, or as a tea (steep 1 tsp of seeds in hot water for 10–15 minutes).
- Bonus: Celery seed extract is also available in supplement form.

Pro Tips:

- Wash well: Celery is on the Dirty Dozen list—opt for organic if possible or wash thoroughly.
- Pair with fat: To better absorb the antioxidants, eat with a healthy fat like olive oil or nuts.

Rosemary

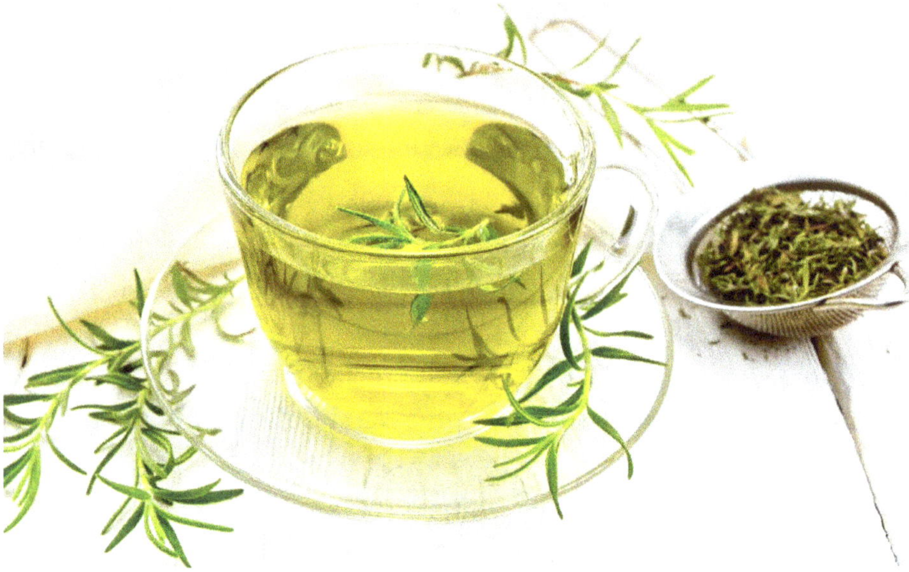

Rosemary isn't just for seasoning your Sunday chicken — it's a serious herb with healing power. Here's why rosemary is a must-have in your herbal toolkit.

Rosemary tea may have many health benefits, including reducing stress and anxiety, improving memory, and supporting digestion.

Potential benefits

- **Antioxidants**: Rosemary tea contains antioxidants that may reduce cell damage.

- **Anti-inflammatory**: Rosemary tea may help relieve muscle pain, joint inflammation, and headaches.

- **Digestion**: Rosemary tea may help with digestive issues like gas, bloating, and indigestion.

- **Immune system**: Rosemary tea may support immune system functions.
- **Hair growth**: Rosemary tea may stimulate hair growth by increasing blood circulation.

- **Eye health**: Rosemary tea may protect against macular degeneration and other eye diseases.

- **Mental concentration:** Rosemary tea may improve mental concentration.

- **Stress and anxiety:** Rosemary tea may have mild calming properties that help relieve stress and anxiety.

Other Uses

Rosemary tea may also help with headaches, fatigue, and stomach upsets.

Rosemary has a long history of culinary and aromatic uses, in addition to applications in traditional herbal and Ayurvedic medicine.

The rosemary bush (Rosmarinus officinalis) is native to South America and the Mediterranean region. It's part of the Lamiaceae family of plants, along with mint, oregano, lemon balm, and basil.

Many people enjoy rosemary tea for its flavor, aroma, and health benefits.

Making rosemary tea is super easy and a great way to enjoy the herb's health benefits. It has a piney, slightly minty flavor and is often used to boost memory, aid digestion, and reduce inflammation.

Here's a simple method:

How to Make Rosemary Tea

Ingredients:

- 1 tsp dried rosemary or 1 fresh rosemary sprig (about 1-2 inches long)
- 1 cup (240 ml) boiling water
- Optional: honey, lemon, or ginger for flavor

Instructions:

1. Boil the water – Bring 1 cup of water to a boil.
2. Add rosemary – Place the dried or fresh rosemary into a teacup or teapot.
3. Pour and steep – Pour the hot water over the rosemary. Cover and let it steep for 5–10 minutes depending on how strong you like it.
4. Strain – Remove the rosemary using a strainer or just lift the sprig out.
5. Sweeten (optional) – Add honey, a squeeze of lemon, or some fresh ginger if desired.

Orange Peel Tea

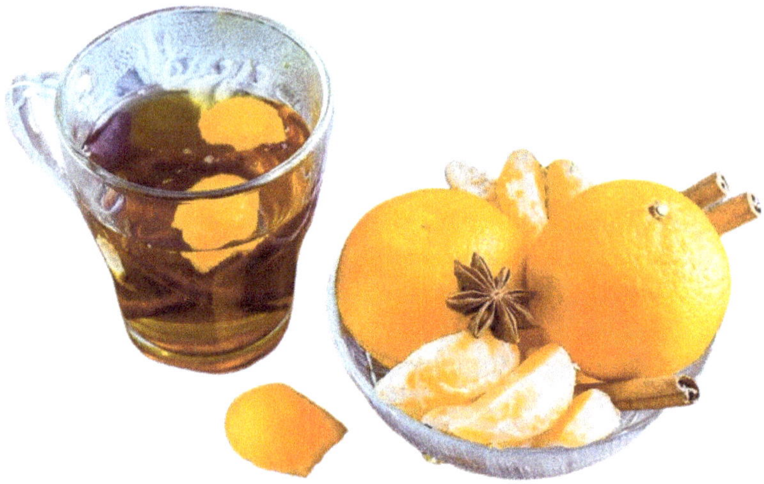

Orange peel tea is rich in vitamin C and flavonoids, which have antioxidant properties that can strengthen the immune system and help to prevent diseases like cancer, high blood pressure, diabetes and the flu.

Orange peel tea is also a great weight loss option, as it has excellent amounts of potassium. This mineral contains diuretic properties that help to eliminate excess body fluid and reduce abdominal bloating.

This tea is prepared using fresh or dried orange peel and can be consumed on its own or flavored with cinnamon, ginger and honey. In order to obtain the health benefits of this tea, it should be incorporated into a healthy, active lifestyle

1. Helping with weight loss

Because it contains excellent amounts of potassium, orange peel tea promotes the elimination of excess body fluid, which can reduce abdominal bloating and contribute to weight loss.

In addition, the peel of the orange contains four times more fiber than the actual fruit, making this tea a good option to help prolong satiety and manage urges to eat.

2. Preventing cancer

Orange peel tea is rich in vitamin C and flavonoids such as hesperidin and naringenin. These have antioxidant action that help to fight excess free radicals and thus prevent some types of cancer.

3. Treating varicose veins

Orange peel has excellent amounts of hesperidin, a flavonoid with anti-inflammatory and antioxidant properties which improve blood circulation.
For this reason, orange peel tea can be a great option for preventing and helping to treat varicose veins and fatigued legs.

4. Controlling high blood pressure

Orange peel tea has excellent amounts of potassium, a mineral that helps to eliminate excess sodium in the body through the urine. This can play a role in managing high blood pressure.

In addition, orange peel contains excellent amounts of antioxidants, such as hesperidin and nobiletin, which improve arterial health and prevent the formation of free radicals, which also contribute to hypertension.

5. Preventing colds and flu

Because it contains three times more vitamin C than the fruit, orange peel tea helps to boost immunity and prevent viral infections.
The antioxidants in orange peels (like hesperidin, nobiletin and naringenin) and also present in high concentrations, making this tea a good option for fighting circulating free radicals and preventing the flu.

6. Preventing neurodegenerative diseases

Orange peel tea contains high levels of the nobiletin and tangeretin, which are flavonoids with anti-inflammatory and antioxidant functions. These can protect central nervous system cells from free radicals, which can help prevent diseases such as dementia, Alzheimer's and Parkinson's disease.

7. Preventing diabetes

Because it contains excellent amounts of antioxidants, orange peel tea helps improve the function of insulin, the hormone responsible for controlling blood sugar levels. Therefore this tea can play a role in preventing diabetes.

8. Detoxing the liver

Orange tea has anti-inflammatory and antioxidant properties, which fight free radicals, as well as protect and improve liver function. This tea has the ability to aid in eliminating toxins from the body.

How to Make Orange Peel Tea

Ingredients:

- 1 tablespoon dried orange peel (or fresh peel, sliced thin)
- 1–2 cups of water
- Honey or lemon (optional)

Boil the Water:

- Bring 1–2 cups of water to a boil in a pot.
- Add the Orange Peel:
- Add the orange peel to the boiling water.
- Reduce the heat and let it simmer for 5–10 minutes.

Strain:

- Pour the tea through a strainer into a cup.
- Add Extras (Optional):
- Sweeten with honey or add a squeeze of lemon for extra flavor.

Enjoy:

Sip and relax — it's great for digestion, stress relief, and immunity!

Tip:

You can store dried orange peels in an airtight jar for future use.

St. John's Wort

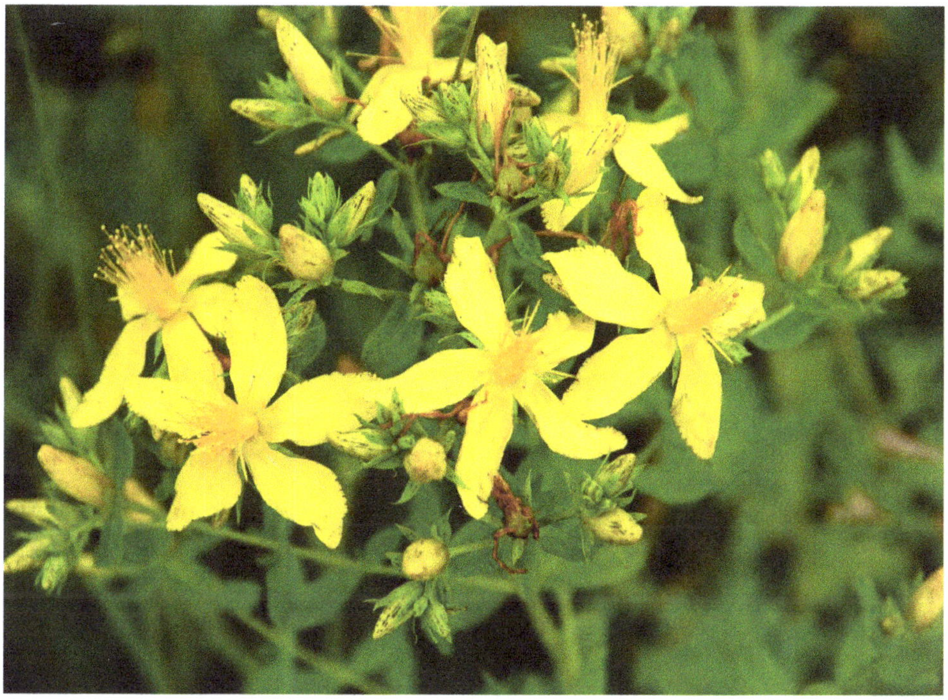

St. John's wort (Hypericum perforatum) has a history of use as a medicine dating back to ancient Greece, where it was used for a range of illnesses, including various nervous disorders. St. John's wort also has antibacterial, antioxidant, and antiviral properties. Because of its anti-inflammatory properties, it has been applied to the skin to help heal wounds and burns.

St. John's wort is one of the most commonly purchased herbal products in the United States.

In recent years, St. John's wort has been studied extensively as a treatment for depression. Most studies show that St. John's wort may help treat mild-to-moderate depression, and has fewer side effects than most other prescription antidepressants. But it interacts with a number of medications, so it should be taken only under the guidance of a health care provider.

Depression

There is good evidence that St. John's wort may reduce symptoms in people with mild-to-moderate, but not severe (or major) depression. In many studies it seems to work as well as selective serotonin reuptake inhibitors (SSRIs), a popular type of antidepressant often prescribed to treat depression. SSRIs include fluoxetine (Prozac), citalopram (Celexa), and sertraline (Zoloft). In addition, St. John's wort doesn't seem to cause loss of sex drive, one of the most common side effects of antidepressants.

Other Uses

St. John's wort has also shown promise in treating the following conditions, a few of which are related to depression.

- **Premenstrual syndrome (PMS)**. Research suggests that St. John's wort may help relieve physical and emotional symptoms of PMS in some women, including cramps, irritability, food cravings, and breast tenderness. One study reported a 50% reduction in symptom severity.

- **Menopause**. There's some evidence to suggest that St. John's wort, combined with black cohosh, helps improve mood and anxiety during menopause.

- **Seasonal affective disorder (SAD).** Used alone, St. John's wort has improved mood in people with SAD, a type of depression that occurs during the winter months because of lack of sunlight. SAD is usually treated with light therapy. Research shows that using St. John's wort together with phototherapy works even better.

Eczema, wounds, minor burns, hemorrhoids. St. John's wort has antibacterial properties and may also help fight inflammation. Applied topically (to the skin), it may relieve symptoms associated with minor wounds and skin irritation.
Obsessive compulsive disorder (OCD), social phobia. One early open-label study found that taking St. John's wort 450 mg, 2 times a day for 12 weeks improved OCD symptoms. However, other studies show that St. John's wort doesn't improve OCD.

Pediatric

Most studies on St. John's wort have been conducted in adults. However, one study (more than 100 children under age 12) indicated that St. John's wort may be a safe and effective way of treating mild-to-moderate symptoms of depression in children.

Never give your child St. John's wort without medical supervision. Children who are being treated with St. John's wort should be carefully monitored for side effects, such as allergic reactions or upset stomach. You should not try to treat depression in a child without a doctor's help because depression can be a serious illness.

Adult

Dry herb (in capsules or tablets). The usual dose for mild depression and mood disorders is 300 mg (standardized to 0.3% hypericin extract), 3 times per day, with meals. St. John's wort is available in time-release capsules.

St. John's wort is also available as a liquid extract or tea. Ask your doctor to help you find the right dose.

It may take 3 to 6 weeks to feel any effects from St. John's wort.

DO NOT stop taking St. John's wort all at once because that may cause unpleasant side effects. Gradually lower the dose before stopping.

How to Make St. John's Wort Tea

You'll Need:

- 1–2 teaspoons of dried St. John's Wort flowers (or a few fresh sprigs if available)
- 1 cup hot water (just below boiling)
- Optional: honey, lemon, or lavender for added flavor and calm

Instructions:

1. Place the dried herb in a cup or teapot.
2. Pour hot water over it.
3. Cover and steep for 10–15 minutes.
4. Strain, then add honey or lemon if desired.
5. Drink 1 cup daily, usually in the evening for relaxation.

Prunella Vulgaris

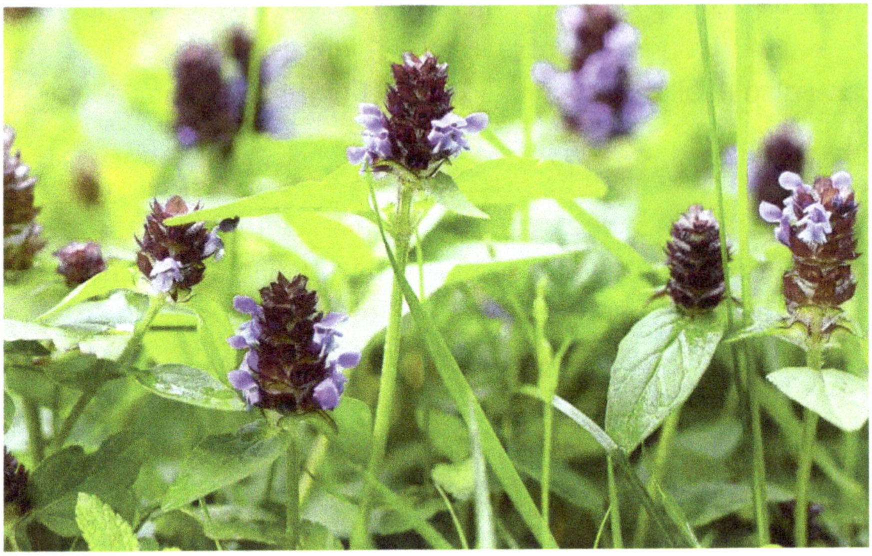

What is Prunella vulgaris?

Prunella vulgaris is an herb that has been used to treat illnesses for centuries. It's a member of the mint family and has large green leaves and purple flowers. It grows all over the world, including North America, Europe, and Asia. Prunella vulgaris is also known as "heal-all" due to its traditional use in healing wounds, throat infections, and several other ailments.

The possible health benefits of this plant are attributed to several of its compounds. These include flavonoids, tannins, and ursolic, rosmarinic, and oleanolic acids, which may have anti-inflammatory and antioxidant properties.

Specifically, these compounds may help prevent complications associated with diabetes, protect against herpes, and have anticancer effects.

All parts of the herb are edible, and you can add its leaves to salads or other recipes.

It's also sold in pill and liquid-extract form, as well as in balms and ointments that can be applied directly to your skin. You can find it online or in supplement shops.

May have cancer-fighting properties

Certain compounds in Prunella vulgaris may have anticancer effects.

Specific carbohydrates in the plant have been shown to induce cancer cell death and prevent tumor growth in test-tube studies.

Test-tube studies also show that caffeic acid, rosmarinic acid, and other plant compounds in this herb may act as antioxidants that fight underlying cell damage.

This damage is caused by reactive molecules called free radicals, which are linked to cancer development.

One study in human liver cancer cells found that Prunella vulgaris stopped the spread of cancer by inhibiting certain enzymes that promote cancer growth.
Furthermore, a study in 424 people with breast cancer found that those who took the herb along with an anticancer medication lived significantly longer than those who took the medication alone.

In fact, almost twice as many people in the group who took Prunella vulgaris with medication showed no evidence of disease after their treatment, compared with the group who did not take the supplement alongside their medication.
However, keep in mind that this research is in its early stages. More human research is needed to fully understand the role of Prunella vulgaris as a complementary cancer therapy.

1. Herbal Tea

Ingredients:

- 1–2 teaspoons dried Prunella vulgaris
- 1 cup hot water

Instructions:

- Add the dried herb to hot water and let it steep for 10–15 minutes.
- Strain and drink warm.
- You can sweeten with honey or add lemon for flavor.

Benefits:

- Great for sore throat, boosting immunity, and general detox.

2. Tincture

- You can purchase Prunella tincture or make your own by soaking the herb in alcohol for 4–6 weeks.
- Take 10–20 drops in water, 1–2 times daily.

Benefits:

- Quick absorption and useful for inflammation, cold sores, and stress relief.

Peppermint

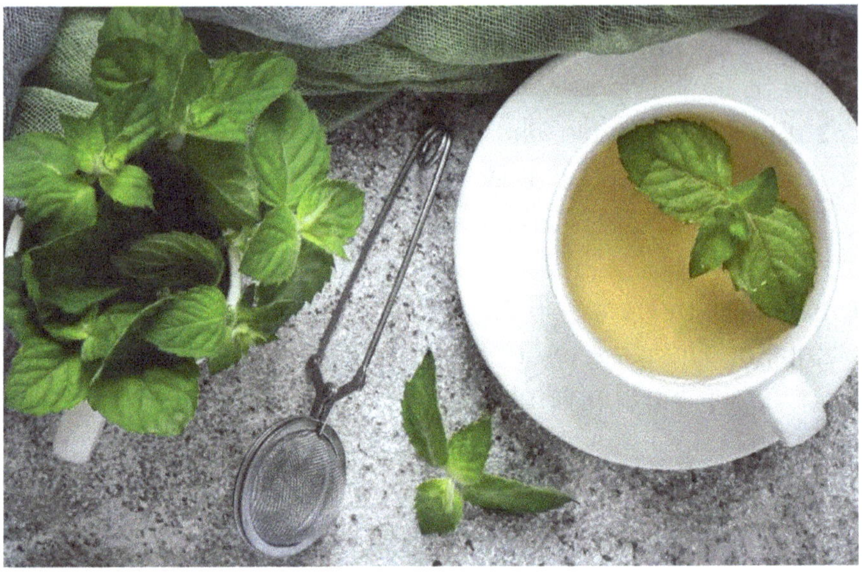

Peppermint tea is naturally sweet and free of caffeine. It may be linked to health benefits, including improving digestion, boosting focus, and relieving migraine. Peppermint (Mentha × piperita) is an aromatic herb in the mint family that is a cross between watermint and spearmint.

Native to Europe and Asia, it has been used for thousands of years for its pleasant, minty taste and health benefits.
Peppermint is used as a flavoring in breath mints, candies, and other foods. Additionally, many people consume peppermint as a refreshing, caffeine-free tea.
Peppermint leaves contain several essential oils including menthol, menthone, and limonene.

Menthol gives peppermint its cooling properties and recognizably minty scent.
While peppermint tea is often drunk for its flavor, it may also have several health benefits.
The tea itself has rarely been studied scientifically, but peppermint extracts have.

May ease digestive issues

Peppermint may relieve digestive symptoms, such as gas, bloating, and indigestion.
Animal studies indicate that peppermint relaxes your digestive system and may ease pain. It also prevents smooth muscles from contracting, which could relieve spasms in your gut.

May help relieve tension headaches and migraines

As peppermint acts as a muscle relaxant and pain reliever, it may diminish certain types of headaches. The menthol in peppermint oil increases blood flow and provides a cooling sensation, possibly easing pain. In one 2010 randomized clinical study in 35 people with migraines, peppermint oil applied to the forehead and temples significantly reduced pain after 2 hours, compared to a placebo.

Another study found that administering peppermint oil drops into the nose reduced the intensity and frequency of headaches and was as effective as lidocaine, a common pain reliever. While the aroma of peppermint tea may help relax muscles and improve headache pain, there is no supporting scientific evidence to confirm this effect. However, applying peppermint oil to your temples may help.

May freshen your breath

There's a reason why peppermint is a common flavoring for toothpastes, mouthwashes, and chewing gums.

In addition to its pleasant smell, peppermint has antibacterial properties that help kill germs that cause dental plaque, which may improve your breath.

In one study, people who had undergone spine surgery and had received a rinse made with peppermint, tea tree, and lemon oils experienced improvement in bad breath symptoms compared to those who did not receive the oils.

In another 2013 study, female students given a peppermint mouth rinse experienced an improvement in breath after 1 week, compared to the control group.

While there is no evidence from scientific studies that drinking peppermint tea has the same effect, the compounds in peppermint have been shown to improve breath.

May relieve clogged sinuses

Peppermint has antibacterial, antiviral, and anti-inflammatory properties. Because of this, peppermint tea may alleviate clogged sinuses due to infections, the common cold, and allergies.

Additionally, some older research demonstrates that menthol — one of the active compounds in peppermint — improves the perception of airflow in your nasal cavity. Therefore, steam from peppermint tea may help you feel as though your breathing is easier.

May improve energy

Peppermint tea may improve energy levels and reduce fatigue.

While there are no studies on peppermint tea specifically, research demonstrates that natural compounds in peppermint may have beneficial effects on energy.

In one study, 24 healthy young people experienced less mental fatigue during a cognitive test when given peppermint oil capsules.

In another study, peppermint oil aromatherapy was found to reduce the incidence of fatigue more effectively than a placebo in people admitted to a cardiology center

Making peppermint tea is super easy and refreshing! Here's a simple way to make it, whether you're using fresh leaves or dried:

Using Fresh Peppermint Leaves

Ingredients:

- A handful of fresh peppermint leaves (about 1/4 cup)
- 2 cups of water
- Honey or sweetener (optional)
- Lemon (optional)

Steps:

1. Rinse the peppermint leaves to clean off any dirt.
2. Boil the 2 cups of water in a kettle or saucepan.
3. Once boiling, remove from heat and add the peppermint leaves.
4. Cover and steep for 5–10 minutes, depending on how strong you like it.
5. Strain the tea into your cup.
6. Add honey or lemon if you like, and enjoy!

Pot Marigold

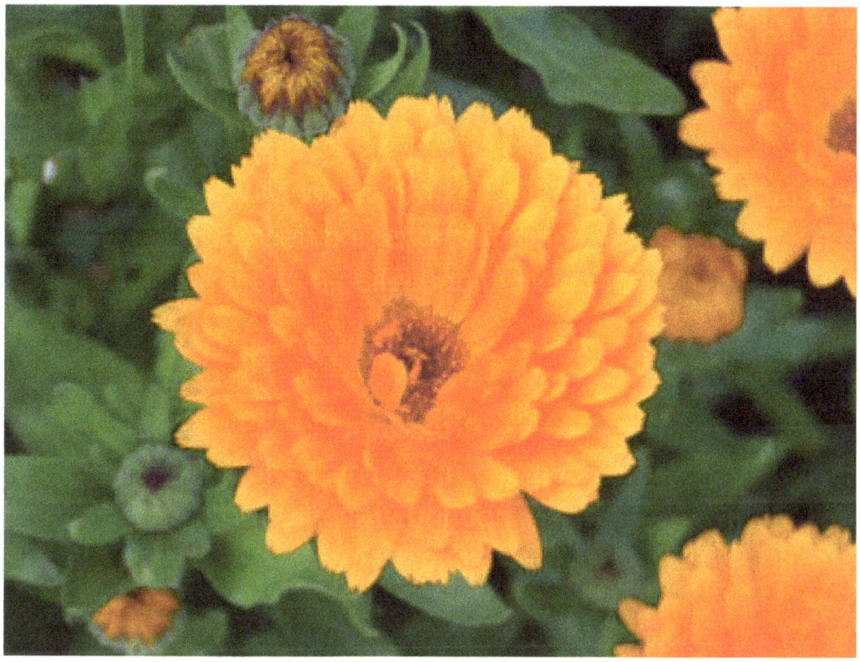

Marigold petals have been used for medicinal purposes since ancient times, including by the Egyptians, Greeks and Romans. Marigold petals were used to treat a variety of health problems, such as stomach aches, menstrual pain and skin inflammation.

Benefits

Skin Healing

Calendula's most popular use from ancient times to modern day has been for healing the skin of wounds, burns, rashes, itchiness, bites and swelling. It has been found that Marigold has the ability to promote the growth of healthy new tissue, increase blood flow to the affected area, boost collagen production (which firms and strengthens skin), hydrate dry skin and speed up the process of skin repair following surgery or damage.

Marigold's ability to help treat wounds is believed to be due to stimulation of epithelial cell production (the cells that make up the outer surface of the body), mostly as a result of the presence of glycoproteins and nucleoproteins. It's also linked to increased cell turnover and improved collagen metabolism stimulation.

Natural Antiseptic/Anti-Inflammatory

Used during First World War and the American Civil War as an antiseptic for wounds, the main compounds within Calendula are the triterpenoids, which are claimed to be the most important anti-inflammatory and anti-edematous (preventing swelling) components within the plant.

Another well-researched use of Marigold extract is applying it in drop form to the inside of the ear canal to help treat bacterial ear infections and decrease pain. It has been found that these drops can lower inner-ear swelling and inflammation within just a couple of days of use.

Antioxidant

Calendula oil is an excellent antioxidant source. This beautiful orange and yellow oil is rich in carotenes and carotenoids - the compounds responsible for the plant's radiant colour. These phytochemicals are pre-cursors to the production of antioxidant Vitamin A.

Conjunctivitis/Eye Inflammation

Research has found that Calendula extract is effective in the treatment of conjunctivitis and other ocular inflammatory conditions. The extract demonstrates antibacterial, anti-viral, antifungal and immuno-stimulating properties that were shown to reduce eye infections. The vision is also protected by these extracts, guarding the delicate tissues of the eye from UV and oxidative damage.

Using Dried or fresh Marigold (Calendula) Petals

Ingredients:

- 1–2 teaspoons dried marigold petals (calendula officinalis)
- 1 cup boiling water
- Honey or lemon (optional)

Steps:

1. Boil water — bring about 1 cup to a rolling boil.
2. Add marigold petals to a tea infuser, teapot, or directly into your cup.
3. Pour the boiling water over the petals.
4. Cover and steep for 10–15 minutes (longer for a stronger brew).
5. Strain the tea if you added petals directly into your cup.
6. Add honey or lemon if desired, and enjoy!

Noni Fruit

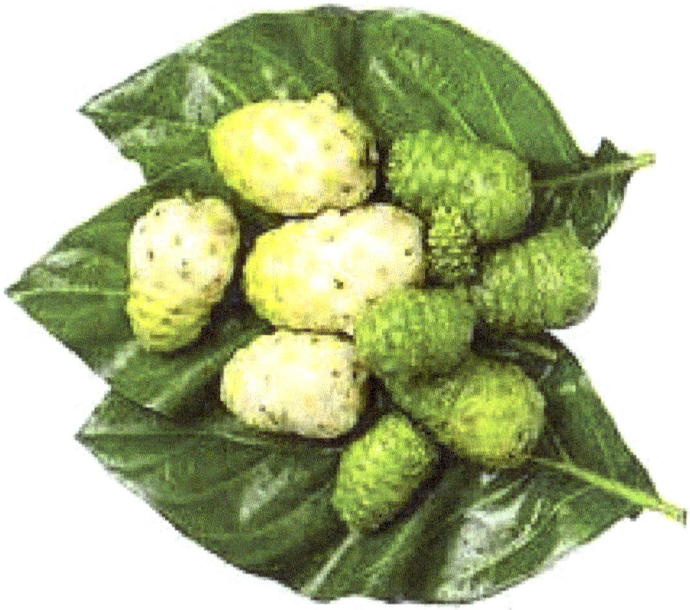

Noni juice is made from the fruit of the noni plant, which is a small evergreen tree in the coffee family that grows in the Pacific Islands, Southeast Asia, Australia, Jamaica and India. It usually grows near lava flows.
Some of the common names around the world for noni include.

- Indian mulberry
- Beach mulberry
- Great morinda
- Headache tree
- Cheese fruit

Noni fruit, leaves, flowers, bark, stems, and roots are used to make dye as well as medicine. Noni juice is made like most juices — from pressing the berries and combining the juices with water and sometimes with sweeteners. This juice has been popular in traditional medicine around the world for many years, and people drink noni juice to help with a variety of ailments like general aches and pains, arthritis, constipation, and infections.

While some scientific evidence supports the claims of health benefits from noni juice, more human research is needed to consider juices from different sources and in broader populations.

Health Benefits

Many of the perceived health benefits of noni juice are not supported by adequate scientific research. However, there is data to suggest that drinking noni juice can:

Reduce Neck Pain

Research shows that drinking noni juice can play a role in treating degenerative musculoskeletal conditions.

In one study, people with age-related spinal damage (cervical osteoarthritis or cervical spondylosis) reported less neck pain and stiffness when they combined noni juice with selected physiotherapies. However, treatment with physiotherapy alone does a better job of relieving pain and improving flexibility than noni juice alone.

Making noni juice at home is pretty straightforward, especially if you've got access to fresh noni fruit. It's known for its strong smell and taste, but also for its many health benefits—immune support, detox, anti-inflammatory, and more. Here's how to do it:

Basic Noni Juice (Fermented Method – Traditional)

Ingredients:

- Ripe noni fruits (soft, translucent, and slightly yellowish)
- A clean glass jar with a lid
- Strainer
- Container for collecting juice

Steps:

1. Wash the noni fruits thoroughly.
2. Place them whole into the clean jar (don't cut them—just pack them in).
3. Cover the jar with the lid loosely (to let gases escape) or use a cloth secured with a rubber band.
4. Let it sit at room temperature, out of direct sunlight, for 2 to 6 weeks.
5. Over time, the fruit will start to ferment and juice will collect at the bottom.
6. Once enough juice has collected, strain it into a clean bottle or jar.
7. Store the juice in the refrigerator. It can last for months when stored properly.

Tip: The longer you ferment, the stronger and more potent the juice.

Lemongrass

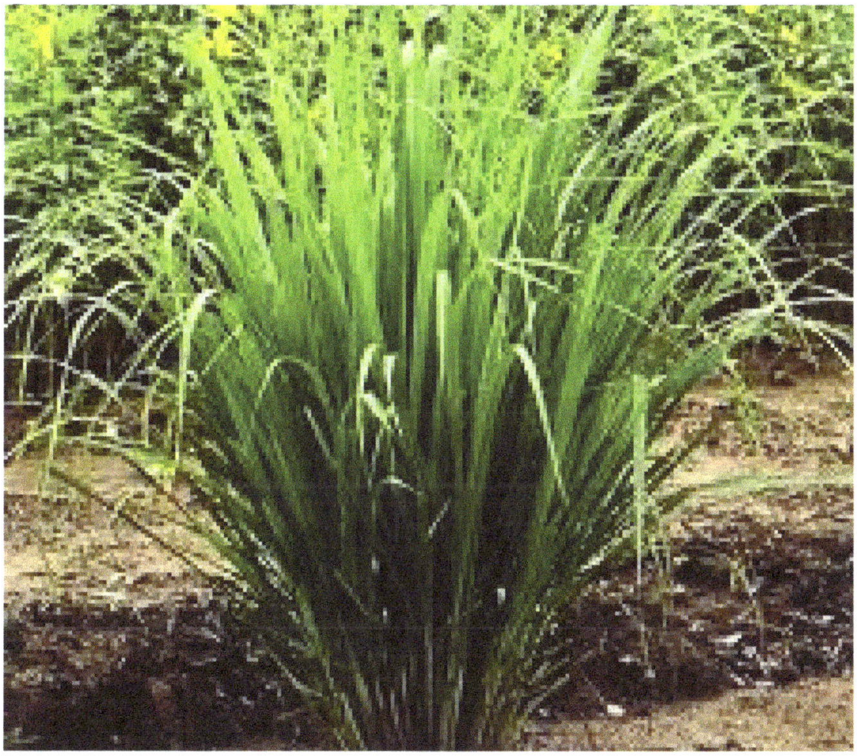

Doctors do know that lemongrass contains the inflammation-fighting compounds chlorogenic acid, isoorientin, and swertiajaponin.
Chronic inflammation is a factor in many adverse health conditions, including diabetes and heart disease. As such, lemongrass tea could be a beneficial drink for people to incorporate into their diet.
Below are five additional health benefits that may result from drinking lemongrass tea.

Many people find sipping hot tea relaxing, but lemongrass tea may offer further anxiety-reducing properties.
Indeed, older research suggests that inhaling lemongrass essential oil may have a calming effect and relieve anxiety.

Lemongrass is a rich source of flavonoids and phenolic compounds, which contain antioxidants. It's also an effective antibacterial and antifungal agent that contains anti-inflammatory and antioxidant properties. Lemongrass contains quercetin, a flavonoid known for having antioxidant and anti-inflammatory benefits.

Top Benefits of Lemongrass Tea

1. Reduces Fever & Cold Symptoms

- Known as "fever grass" for a reason
- Helps sweat out fever and ease sore throat or cough

2. Lowers Blood Pressure

- Acts as a natural diuretic, reducing water retention
- May help relax blood vessels, supporting heart health

3. Relieves Stress & Anxiety

- Natural calming effect on the nervous system
- Great as an evening tea to unwind and improve sleep

4. Aids Digestion

- Reduces bloating, gas, and stomach cramps
- Stimulates bowel movement and helps relieve constipation

5. Detoxifies the Body

- Supports liver and kidney function
- Helps flush out toxins and cleanse the system

6. Boosts Immunity

- Rich in antioxidants, vitamin C, and antimicrobial compounds
- Helps fight infections and strengthen overall immune function

7. Anti-inflammatory & Pain Relief

- May help relieve joint pain, headaches, and menstrual cramps

8. Anticancer properties

- Some studies suggest that lemongrass may have anticancer properties.
- According to a 2021 review, lemongrass oil contains a compound called citral, which shows promise in stopping the growth of various cancer cells, including prostate, breast, ovarian, and lung cancers. It is thought to specifically target cancer cells without harming normal cells.

Lemongrass tea recipe

It is possible to make lemongrass tea at home. After purchasing the stalks at a grocery store or herbalist, people can take the following steps to brew their tea:

- use 1-2 stalks cut into 1- to 2-inch pieces
- boil a cup of water
- pour the boiling water over the lemongrass stalks to steep
- leave the stalks in the water for at least 5 minutes
- strain the liquid from the stalks and pour into a teacup
- Adding ice cubes will create a cold lemongrass tea.

The tea should have a fresh, citrusy taste. A person could start with one cup of lemongrass tea per day, then add more to their diet over the next days if they wish to. Alternatively, most grocery and health food stores sell lemongrass tea.

Callaloo

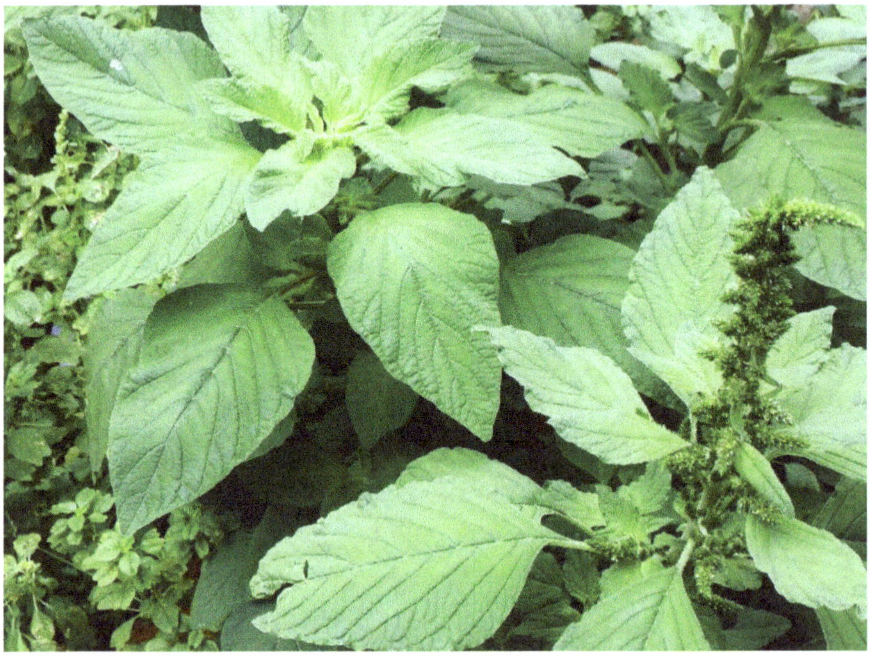

Health Benefits of Jamaican Callaloo / Amaranth Greens.
The herbal plant called Callaloo is the popular Jamaican name for what is otherwise known as Amaranth greens. The scientific name of the plant is Amaranthus spinosus or Amaranth.

Nutritional Values in Callaloo

Due to its high content of vitamin A and C, which produces antioxidants, callaloo is great in treating inflammation, ulcers and irritations of both the external and internal organs. For example this herb may be applied to the skin to treat bruises and also used as a gargle for throat irritations, or simply used as a mouthwash.

Some of the nutrients in callaloo are better retrieved in raw form, such as vitamin C which can be added to the diet through juicing.

Some Minerals found in Callaloo are: Iron, calcium, vitamin A, vitamin b and vitamin c, protein, fiber, magnesium, potassium etc.

Seven (7) Health Benefits of Callaloo

- Potassium in callaloo improves and maintains cardiovascular health by reducing blood clots and helping to maintain a steady blood pressure flow.

- Great in balancing digestive health due to fiber content- fiber is the roughage that helps to clean up the intestinal tracts, creating a feeling of lightness while eliminating toxic waste from the body.

- Great for the blood and red blood cell growth by the presence of iron in the leafy greens.

- Improves and maintains bone and teeth health from the calcium that is found in most leafy greens.

- Hair and skin benefits well from this herb, improving conditions of unwanted graying and promoting glowing skin.

- Vitamin C helps to boost the immune system, protecting the body from surrounding ailments.

- Overall vibrancy. Callaloo greens packs so many nutrients and minerals that aids in the functioning of our body systems, such as the digestive tract, and keeps the body in good tip top shape.

Callaloo is a leafy green that's typically cooked by steaming it with vegetables and seasonings. You can use fresh or canned callaloo.

Ingredients:

- Onion
- Garlic
- Scotch bonnet or hot pepper
- Tomato
- Thyme
- Salt and pepper

Steps

1. Sauté onions in hot oil until softened and translucent
2. Add other vegetables and seasonings
3. Stir in callaloo
4. Cover and steam until tender
5. Optionally, purée until smooth

Papaya Leaf

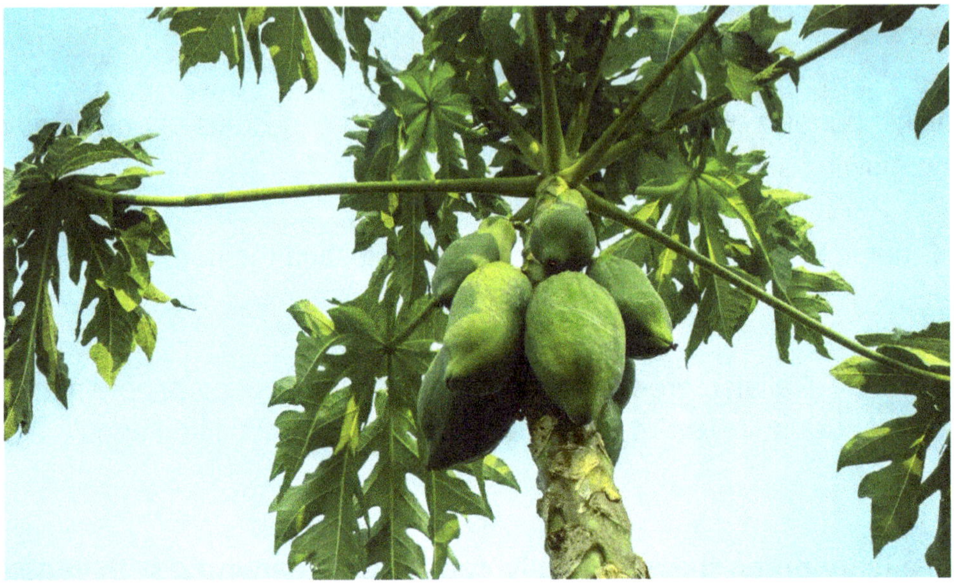

Carica papaya — also simply known as papaya or pawpaw — is a type of tropical, fruit-bearing tree native to Mexico and northern regions of South America. Today, papaya is one of the most widely cultivated crops in the world. Its fruit, seeds, and leaves are frequently utilized in a variety of culinary and folk medicine practices.

Papaya leaf contains unique plant compounds that have demonstrated broad pharmacological potential in test-tube and animal studies.
Although human research is lacking, many papaya leaf preparations, such as teas, extracts, tablets, and juices, are often used to treat illnesses and promote health in numerous ways.
Here are 7 emerging benefits and uses of papaya leaf.

1. May treat symptoms related to dengue fever

One of the most prominent medicinal benefits of papaya leaf is its potential to treat certain symptoms associated with dengue fever.
Dengue is a mosquito-borne virus that can be transmitted to humans and cause flu-like symptoms, such as fever, fatigue, headaches, nausea, vomiting, and skin rashes. Severe cases can also result in reduced platelet levels in the blood. Low platelet levels can contribute to an increased risk of bleeding and are potentially fatal if left untreated.

2. May promote balanced blood sugar

Papaya leaf is often used in Mexican folk medicine as a natural therapy for treating diabetes and improving blood sugar control.

3. May support digestive function

Papaya leaf teas and extracts are often used as an alternative therapy to alleviate uncomfortable digestive symptoms, such as gas, bloating, and heartburn.

Papaya leaf contains fiber — a nutrient that supports healthy digestive function — and a unique compound called papain.

Papain is well known for its ability to break down large proteins into smaller, easier-to-digest proteins and amino acids. It's even used as a meat tenderizer in culinary practices. One study found that the supplemental use of a papain powder sourced from papaya fruit reduced negative digestive symptoms, including constipation and heartburn, in people with irritable bowel syndrome (IBS).

4. May have anti-inflammatory effects

Various papaya leaf preparations are frequently used to remedy a broad range of internal and external inflammatory conditions, including skin rashes, muscle aches, and joint pain.

Papaya leaf contains various nutrients and plant compounds with potential anti-inflammatory benefits, such as papain, flavonoids, and vitamin E.

5. May support hair growth

Topical applications of papaya leaf masks and juices are often used to improve hair growth and scalp health, but evidence to support its efficacy for these purposes is extremely limited.

Some research suggests that high levels of oxidative stress in the body may contribute to hair loss. Eating antioxidant-rich foods may help alleviate oxidative stress and subsequently improve hair growth.

Papaya leaf contains several compounds with antioxidant properties, such as flavonoids and vitamin E.

6. May promote healthy skin

Papaya leaf is frequently consumed orally or applied topically as a way to maintain soft, clear, and youthful-looking skin. A protein-dissolving enzyme in papaya leaf called papain can be used topically as an exfoliant to remove dead skin cells and potentially reduce the occurrence of clogged pores, ingrown hairs, and acne.

Moreover, papaya leaf enzymes have been used to promote wound healing, and one study found they minimized the appearance of scar tissue in rabbits.

7. May have anticancer properties

Papaya leaf has been used in traditional medicine practices to prevent and treat certain types of cancer, but modern research is still lacking.

Papaya leaf extract has demonstrated a powerful ability to inhibit the growth of prostate and breast cancer cells in test-tube studies, but neither animal nor human experiments have replicated these results.

How to Make Papaya Leaf Tea (Fresh Leaves)

Ingredients:

- 1–2 fresh papaya leaves
- 2–3 cups of water
- Honey or lemon (optional, for taste)

Steps:

1. Wash the leaves thoroughly to remove any dirt or residue.
2. Chop the leaves into small pieces.
3. Add them to a saucepan with the water.
4. Bring to a boil, then lower the heat and simmer for 15–20 minutes.
5. Remove from heat and let it cool a bit.
6. Strain into a cup or bottle.
7. Add honey or lemon if the taste is too bitter.

Oregano

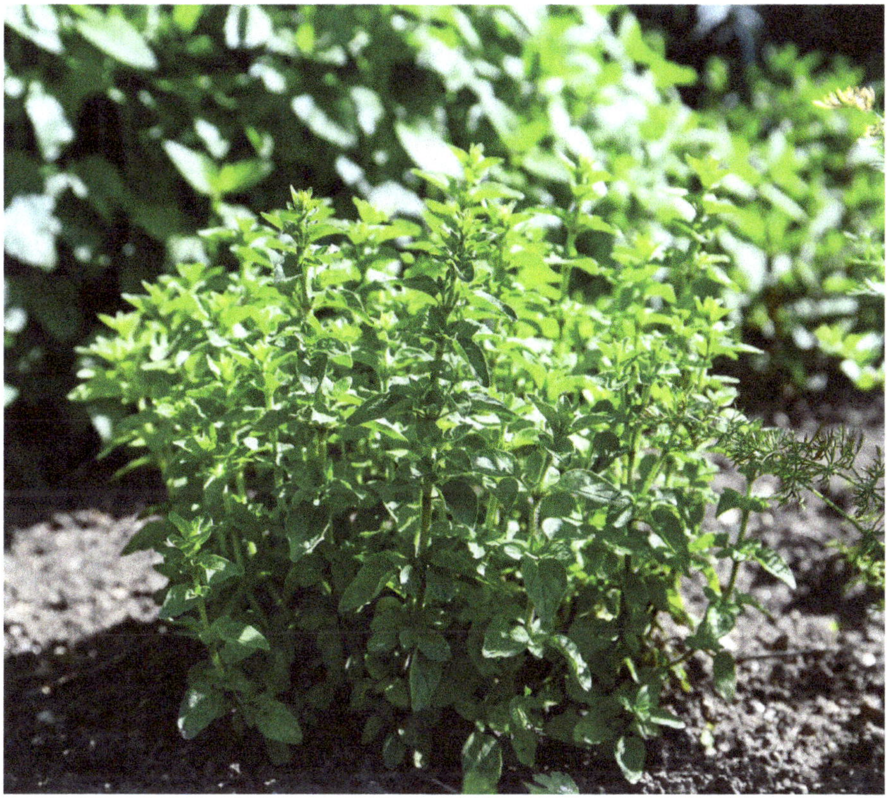

Oregano is a herb packed with antioxidants and antimicrobial properties, making it beneficial for fighting bacteria and inflammation, potentially aiding in digestion, and even helping with respiratory issues like coughs; it's commonly used in cooking to flavor dishes like pizza and pasta, and can also be consumed as a tea or in the form of essential oil.

Key benefits of oregano:

- **Antioxidant power:** Contains high levels of antioxidants like carvacrol and thymol, which can help combat free radical damage in the body.

- **Antimicrobial properties:** May help fight off certain bacteria and fungi due to its active compounds, potentially aiding in treating infections.

- **Anti-inflammatory effects**: Can help reduce inflammation throughout the body.
-
- **Digestive support**: May aid in digestion by reducing bloating and discomfort.
-
- **Respiratory benefits**: Some evidence suggests oregano may help soothe coughs and congestion.

Common uses of oregano:

Culinary:

Adding fresh or dried oregano to dishes like pizza, pasta sauce, tomato-based recipes, grilled meats, and salads.

Tea:

- Brewing oregano leaves into a tea for potential digestive and respiratory benefits.

Essential oil:

- Diluted oregano oil can be used topically for skin concerns or inhaled for aromatherapy.

Important considerations:

Dosage matters:

While oregano is generally safe in culinary amounts, consuming high doses of oregano oil can cause stomach upset.

Consult a healthcare professional:

If you are pregnant, breastfeeding, or have any existing medical conditions, talk to your doctor before using oregano supplements or essential oils.

Marjoram

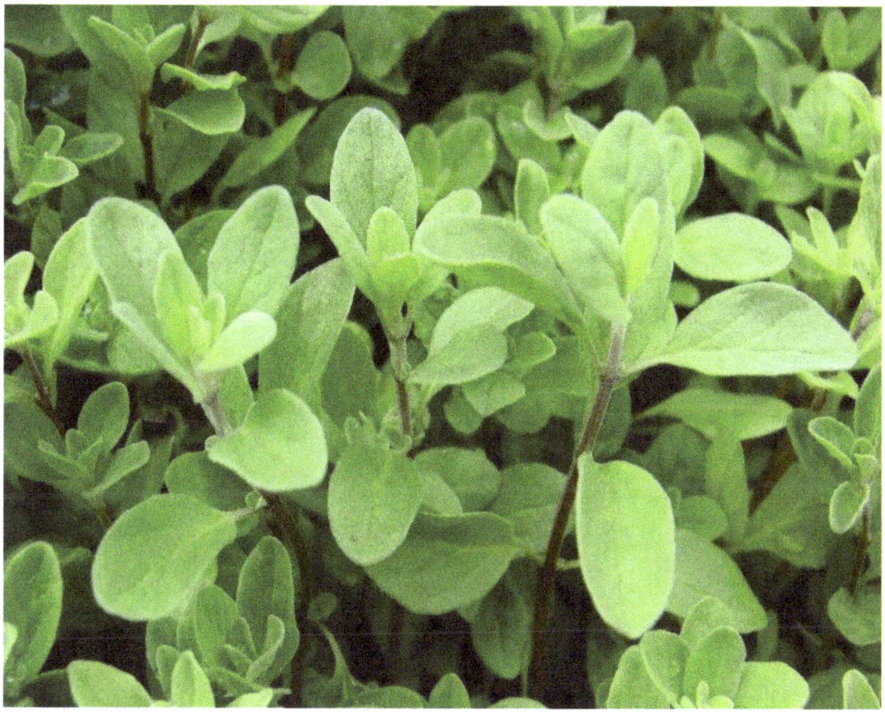

What is marjoram?
Marjoram, also known as sweet marjoram, is an aromatic herb in the mint family that has been grown in the Mediterranean, North Africa, and Western Asia for thousands of years.

While similar to oregano, it has a milder flavor and is often used to garnish salads, soups, and meat dishes.
It's particularly potent when dried but can also be used fresh.

What's more, marjoram has been shown to have several anti-inflammatory and antimicrobial properties. It has been used medicinally to help treat a variety of ailments, including digestive issues, infections, and painful menstruation.
Fresh or dried leaves can be made into a tea or extract. Both forms can be found in health food stores or online.

It's important to note that marjoram extracts vary in strength and purity based on the manufacturer and source. To make sure you're getting a high-quality product, look for third-party certification on the label.

Potential benefits

Research suggests that marjoram may have several health benefits.

Antioxidant and anti-inflammatory properties

Antioxidants help prevent cell damage caused by potentially harmful molecules called free radicals. Several compounds in marjoram, such as carvacrol, have been shown to have antioxidant effects.

In particular, they may help reduce inflammation in your body.

While inflammation is a normal bodily response, chronic inflammation can increase your risk of certain diseases, including diabetes, cancer, and autoimmune disorders.

Thus, reducing inflammation may lower your risk.

May have antimicrobial activity

Marjoram has also demonstrated antimicrobial properties.

Common uses include applying its diluted essential oil to your skin to treat fungal infections, as well as taking supplements to help treat overgrowth of gut bacteria.

Marjoram tea is a gentle, aromatic herbal tea known for its calming effects, helping with digestion, sleep, stress, and even menstrual discomfort. It's super easy to make too!

How to Make Marjoram Tea (Fresh or Dried Leaves)

Ingredients:

- 1 tablespoon fresh marjoram leaves (or 1 teaspoon dried)
- 1 cup boiling water
- Honey or lemon (optional)

Punarnava

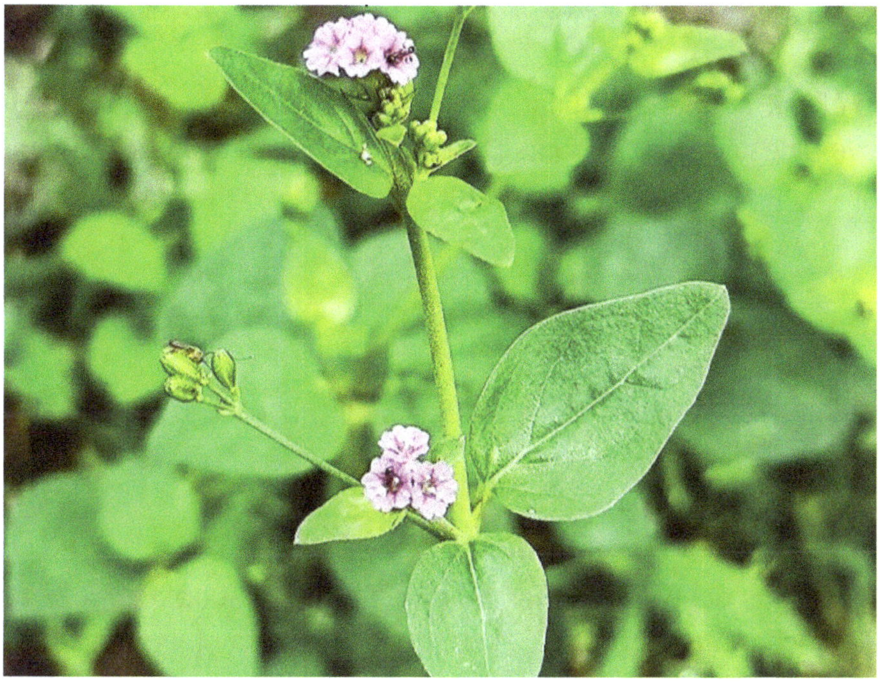

Punarnava is a well known medicinal plant packed with essential nutrients, vitamins such as vitamin C and other constituents.
Taking Punarnava juice before meals might help manage stomach disorders such as constipation by promoting bowel movements due to its laxative property.

It also provides relief from gas and abdominal pain. Punarnava is effective in improving digestion and managing weight by suppressing appetite. Punarnava also helps increase urine production due to its diuretic activity and reduces the risk of urinary complications. It might also be useful for managing liver problems due to its antioxidant activity which prevents liver cell damage caused by free radicals.

Applying Punarnava paste helps to heal skin due to its quick wound healing activity. Moreover, according to Ayurveda, massaging with Punarnava oil helps reduce joint pain due to its Vata balancing property.
It is advisable to use Punarnava powder with water or coconut oil if you have hypersensitive skin.

1. Liver disorders

Punarnava is used to revitalize and clean the liver. According to Ayurveda, when the liver is unable to perform well it also leads to an imbalance of Vata - Pitta-Kapha doshas. This might lead to liver diseases like jaundice. Taking Punanarva helps to correct the function of the liver by removing toxins from the liver cells.

This is because of its Shodhan (purification) and Mutral (diuretic) properties. Punanarva also helps to improve digestive fire due to its Deepan (appetizer) property. It helps to digest the food easily and reduce the burden of liver.

Tips:

a. Take 1-2 teaspoon of Punarnava juice.
b. Add the same quantity of water to it.
c. Have it once or twice a day before taking meals to get rid of the symptoms of liver disorders.

2. Urinary Tract Infection

Urinary tract infection is described under the broad term of Mutrakcchra in Ayurveda. Mutra means ooze, krichra means painful. Thus, dysuria and painful urination are called as Mutrakcchra. In urinary tract infection, Punarnava helps to control burning sensation because it has Mutral (diuretic) effect. It increases the urine flow and subsides the symptoms of UTI like burning sensation during urination.

Tips:

a. Take 1-2 teaspoon of Punarnava juice.
b. Add the same quantity of water to it.
c. Have it once or twice a day before taking meals to get rid of the symptoms of UTI.

3. Obesity

Punarnava is one of the most common herbs which is used to manage weight. An increase in the weight is due to unhealthy food habits and lifestyle which leads to a weak digestive fire. This increases accumulation of Ama causing an imbalance in Meda dhatu and thus resulting in obesity. Punarnava is useful to control obesity as it helps improve metabolism and reduce Ama. This is because of its Deepan (appetizer) and Pachan (digestive) properties. Punarnava also removes excess fluids and waste products from the body by increasing the urine flow due to its Mutral (diuretic) nature.

Tips:

a. Take 1-2 teaspoon of Punarnava juice.
b. Add the same quantity of water to it.
c. Have it once or twice a day before taking meals to get rid of the symptoms of obesity.

4. Rheumatoid Arthritis (RA)

Punarnava helps to reduce the symptoms of rheumatoid arthritis-like pain and swelling. Rheumatoid arthritis (RA) is known as Amavata in Ayurveda. Amavata is a disease in which vitiation of Vata dosha and accumulation of Ama (toxic remains in the body due to improper digestion) takes place in the joints.

Amavata starts with a weak digestive fire which leads to accumulation of Ama. This Ama is carried to different locations through Vata but instead of being absorbed, it gets accumulated in the joints. Punarnava helps to correct digestive fire and reduce Ama due to its Deepan (appetizer) and Pachan (digestive) properties. It also has Vata balancing and Mutral (diuretic) properties which gives relief from the symptoms of Rheumatoid arthritis like pain and swelling in the joints.

Tips:

a. Take 1-2 teaspoon of Punarnava juice.
b. Add the same quantity of water to it.
c. Have it once or twice a day before taking meals to get rid of the symptoms of Rheumatoid arthritis

How to use Punarnava

A. Punarnava Leaf Juice:

a. Take 1-2 teaspoon of Punarnava leaf juice.
b. Add the same quantity of water to it.
c. Take this juice once a day to improve the function of the liver and for fast recovery from jaundice.

B. Punarnava Paste:

a. Take ½ -1 teaspoon of Punarnava root or leave paste.
b. Add cow's milk to it and consume.
c. Use this remedy twice a day to improve the functioning of female reproductive system.

C. Punarnava Churna

a. Take ¼ - ½ teaspoon of Punarnava churna.
b. Add cow's milk or honey to it.
c. Use this remedy once or twice a day to improve the functioning of the male and the female reproductive system.

D. Punarnava Kwath

a. Take 1/2- 1 teaspoon of Punarnava powder.
b. Add 2 cups of water and boil till the volume reduces to 1/2 cup.
c. This is Punarnava Kwath.
d. Take 3-4 teaspoons of this Punarnava Kwath.
e. Add the same quantity of water to it.
f. Drink it preferably once or twice a day to manage jaundice, conjunctivitis.
It is also good to improve the respiratory and urinary system.

Benefits of Punarnava

1. Wound healing

Punarnava helps in quick healing of the wound, decreases swelling and brings back the normal texture of the skin. It helps in quick healing of the wound and reduces inflammation. This is due to its Ropan (healing) property.

Tips:

a. Take 1/2-1 teaspoon of Punaarnava powder or as per your requirement.
b. Make a paste with milk or mustard oil and apply to affected area.
c. Repeat this daily for quick healing of the wound.

2. Joint pain

Punarnava helps to reduce bone and joint pain when applied to the affected area. According to Ayurveda, the bones and joints are considered a site of Vata in the body. Pain in the joints is mainly due to Vata imbalance. Applying or massaging with Punarnava base oil helps to reduce joint pain. This is due to its Vata balancing property.

Tips:

a. Take 1/2-1 teaspoon of Punaarnava powder or as per your requirement.
b. Make a paste with hot water or mustard oil and apply to affected area.
c. Repeat this daily to manage joint pain.

Gymnema

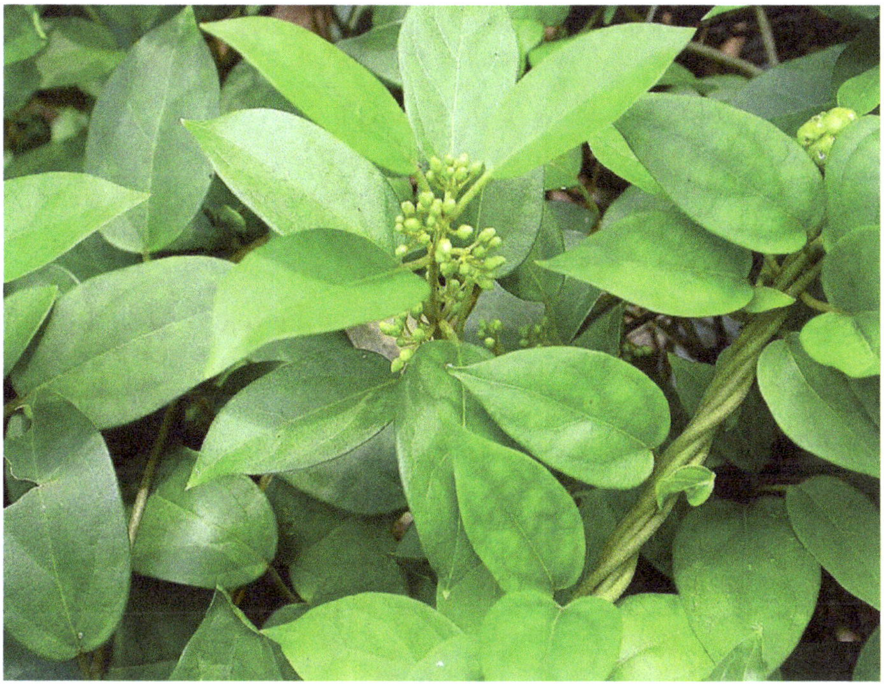

The Gymnema sylvestre plant offers numerous health benefits. For example, it may help you fight sugar cravings and lower high blood sugar levels. It may also help fight inflammation, aid weight loss, and lower "bad" LDL cholesterol and triglyceride levels.

Gymnema sylvestre is a woody climbing shrub that's native to the tropical forests of India, Africa and Australia.
Its leaves have been used in the ancient Indian medicinal practice Ayurveda for thousands of years. It has been a traditional remedy for various ailments, including diabetes, malaria and snakebites.

This herb is thought to inhibit sugar absorption and thus has become a popular study subject in Western medicine.

Gymnema sylvestre can help reduce sugar cravings.
One of the primary active components in this plant is gymnemic acid, which helps suppress sweetness.

When consumed prior to a sugary food or beverage, gymnemic acid blocks the sugar receptors on your taste buds.
Research shows that Gymnema sylvestre extracts can reduce the ability to taste sweetness and thus make sweet foods less appealing.

In a study in fasted individuals, half were given Gymnema extract. Those who received the supplement had less appetite for sweet foods at a subsequent meal and were more likely to limit their food intake, compared to those not taking the extract.

Studies suggest that consuming 200–400 mg of gymnemic acid reduces the intestinal absorption of the sugar glucose.
In one study, Gymnema appeared to improve blood sugar control in people with type 2 diabetes by lowering blood sugar levels.

The study concluded that reducing blood sugar after a meal resulted in a decrease in average blood sugar levels over time. This could help decrease long-term complications of diabetes.

For people with high blood sugar or a high HbA1c, Gymnema sylvestre can help reduce fasting, post-meal and long-term blood sugar levels. However, if you're taking blood-sugar-lowering medications, consult with your doctor first.
Summary

How to Make Gymnema (Gymnia) Tea

Ingredients:

- 1 teaspoon dried Gymnema sylvestre leaves (or 1 tea bag)
- 1 cup hot water (not boiling)
- Optional: cinnamon or ginger (for taste)

Steps:

1. Heat water until just below boiling (about 190–200°F or 88–93°C).
2. Place the dried leaves or tea bag in a cup.
3. Pour the hot water over the leaves.
4. Cover and steep for 5–10 minutes.
5. Strain if using loose leaves.
6. Drink as is, or add a slice of ginger or cinnamon if the taste is too earthy or bitter.

Witch Hazel

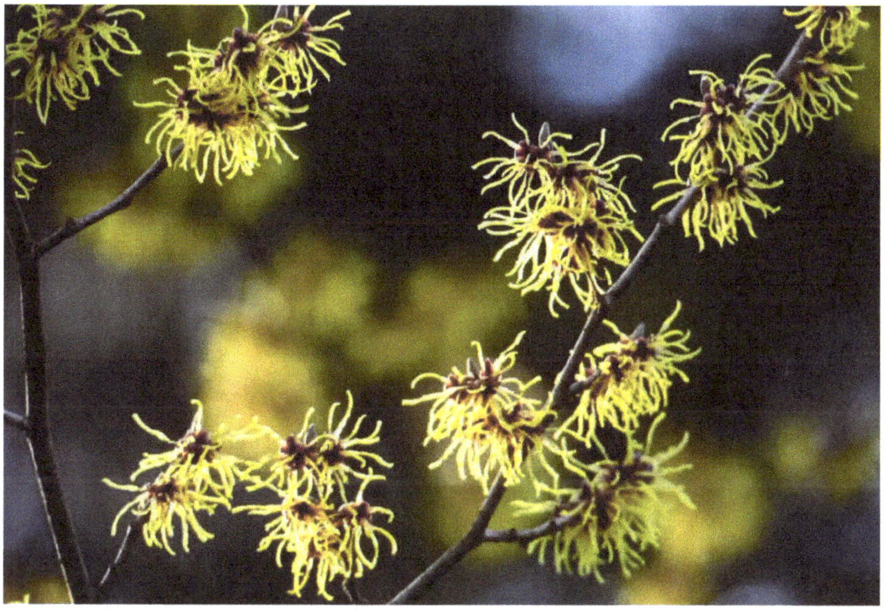

Witch hazel is a widely known plant with a lengthy history of use in the Americas. The plant, including the crude leaf and bark, is used in a variety of forms; fluid extracts, poultices, and most commonly as witch hazel water.

The latter, also known as Hamamelis water or distilled witch hazel extract, is obtained from recently cut, partially dormant twigs. This plant material is soaked in warm water, followed by distillation and the addition of alcohol to the distillate.
Witch hazel water is the most commonly found commercial preparation, usually kept in most homes as a topical cooling agent or astringent.
Traditionally, witch hazel was known to native North American people as a treatment for tumors and eye inflammations.

It was used internally for bleeding. Other uses include treatment of hemorrhoids, burns, cancers, tuberculosis, colds, and fever. Preparations have been used on the skin for treatment of itching and inflammation, as well as in preparations for eye irritation.

- **Acne**: Witch hazel can reduce inflammation and redness.
- **Eczema:** Witch hazel can reduce inflammation and redness.
- **Insect bites:** Witch hazel can soothe minor skin irritations.
- **Bruises and minor burns**: Witch hazel can relieve swelling, bleeding, itching, and minor pain.
- **Varicose veins**: Witch hazel may improve circulation and strengthen venous connective tissue.

Witch hazel has many uses, including as a cleanser, toner, spot treatment, and astringent for the skin and scalp. You can apply it with a cotton ball or pad.

Skin

- **Cleanse oily skin**: Witch hazel's astringent properties help remove excess oil from the skin.
- **Soothe insect bites**: Witch hazel constricts blood vessels to reduce inflammation.
- **Treat acne**: Witch hazel's anti-inflammatory and antibacterial properties help reduce inflammation and fight acne-causing bacteria.
- **Treat puffy eyes**: Witch hazel constricts blood vessels to reduce inflammation.

Witch hazel is a super versatile natural remedy that's been used for centuries. It's a liquid extract from the witch hazel plant (usually Hamamelis virginiana) and is commonly found as a clear astringent in drugstores. You can use it for skin care, soothing irritation, and even minor wounds.
Here's a breakdown of how to use it based on different needs:

For Skin Care (Toner or Astringent)

- Pour some witch hazel on a cotton pad.
- Wipe over your face or oily areas (like forehead, nose, chin).
- Helps to tighten pores, reduce oiliness, and calm inflammation.
- Great for acne-prone skin!
- Use once or twice a day (avoid overuse—it can dry out your skin).

2. For Razor Bumps or Aftershave

- Dab on freshly shaved skin to prevent razor burn and reduce redness.
- It's cooling and helps disinfect small nicks or cuts.

3. For Sunburn or Minor Burns

- Soak a cloth or cotton pad in witch hazel and place it on the affected area.
- It soothes, cools, and reduces swelling.

4. For Bug Bites or Itchy Skin

- Apply directly to bites or itchy patches.
- Helps reduce itching, swelling, and redness.

5. For Hemorrhoids

- Use it on a cotton pad or in a sitz bath.
- Witch hazel is a key ingredient in many hemorrhoid pads and creams.
- It helps reduce swelling and soothe pain.

6. For Bruises or Minor Cuts

- Dab witch hazel on the area with a cotton ball.
- It can help reduce inflammation and speed up healing.

Donkey Pee Pee

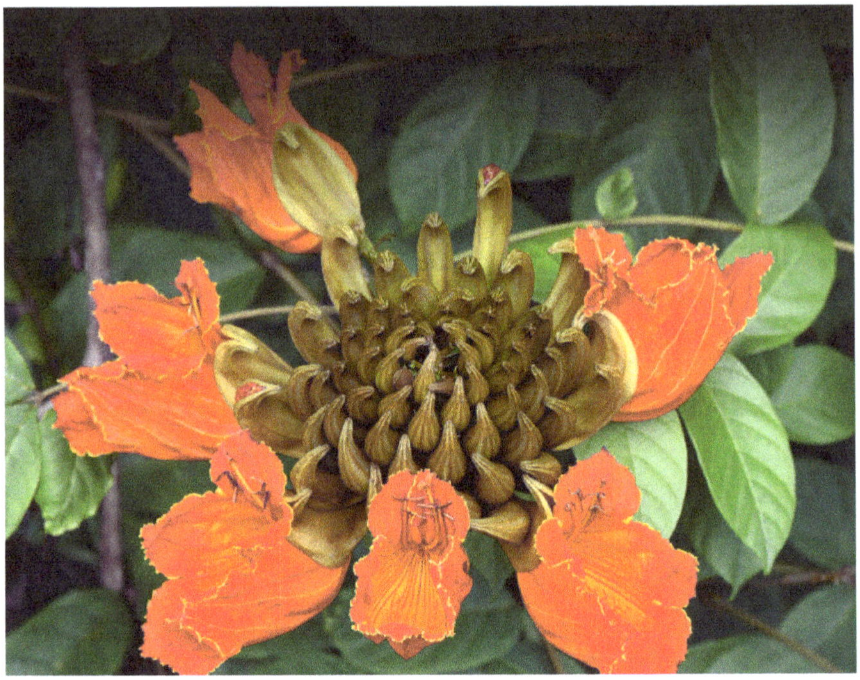

The African Tulip, referred to locally as 'Donkey Pee Pee', has been around for centuries after being brought to Jamaica by West Africans during the Trans-Atlantic slave trade. Locals claimed it can heal all eye conditions including glaucoma.

Besides having a peculiar and rather humorous alias, the plant has been used medicinally as eyedrops by Jamaicans for generations. Its popularity has recently been revived as folks seek natural alternatives for common ailments.

The plant is commonly used as an eyedrop as its spuds store water in preparation for drought.

If someone had an irritated eye, maybe an eye-itch that won't budge, or simply wanted to flush debris out, this plant could do the trick.

Though its medicinal value as an eyedrop has not been proven, the African Tulip has other functions.

According to ScienceDirect.com, the African tulip tree has been used to treat epilepsy and convulsion control, kidney disease and urethritis, and as an antidote for animal poisons. The plant is also reported to exhibit anti-plasmodial and anti-inflammatory properties.

Maybe next time you are out on a stroll in the woods, and there are no water sources close by —- look around for a Donkey pee-pee tree, it may come in handy.

Infusions and decoctions

- Use the bark or leaves to make infusions or decoctions to treat malaria, gastrointestinal issues, and skin conditions.

- Eye drops

- Use the nectar from the flowers as eye drops

- The plant has been used in Jamaica for generations as eyedrops

Laxative

- Use the nectar from the flowers as a mild laxative

- Treat throat irritations

- Other medicinal uses Treat epilepsy, Treat kidney disease, and Use as an antidote for animal poisons.

Jatropha Gossypifolia

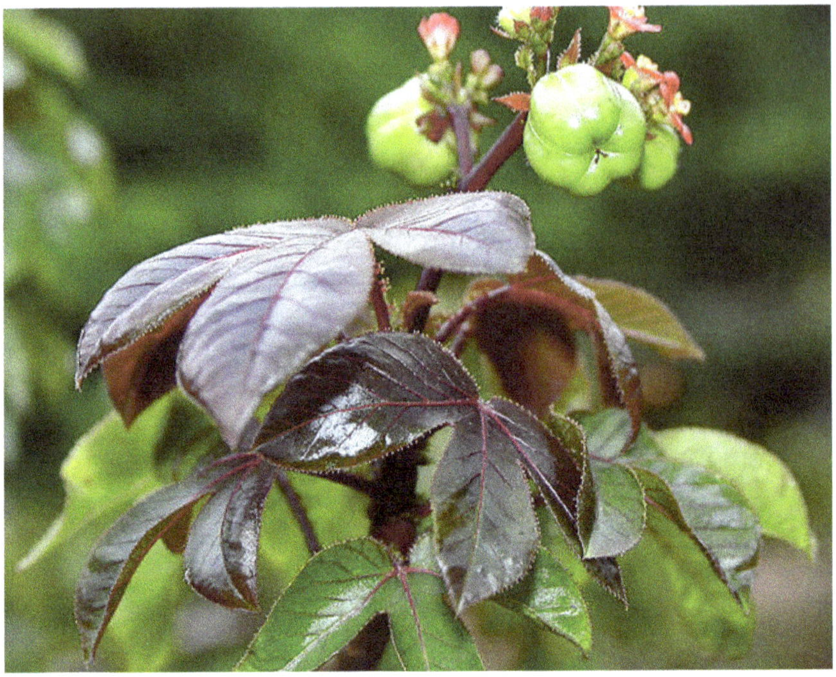

Jatropha gossypiifolia, commonly known as bellyache bush, black physicnut or cotton-leaf physicnut, is a species of flowering plant in the spurge family, Euphorbiaceae. The species is native to Mexico, South America, and the Caribbean islands, but is currently spread throughout the tropics

Jatropha gossypifolia is a medicinal plant used in traditional medicine for many conditions, including fevers, wounds, and inflammation.

Uses

- **Leaves**: Used to treat fevers, eczema, sores, and swollen breasts. Leaf decoctions are used for bathing wounds.
- **Sap:** Used to stop bleeding from the nose, gums, or skin.
- **Root and stem**: Used to treat inflammation and infections.
- **Seeds and fruits:** Used to treat influenza, diarrhea, and as a sedative or analgesic.
- **Latex**: Used to treat wounds and bites from venomous animals.
- **Branches:** Used as a "thick blood" agent.

Other uses

- Used as an oral contraceptive and abortifacient
- Used as a pesticide and insecticide
- Used as a vermifuge

How it's used

Different parts of the plant are used in infusions, decoctions, and macerations.
The plant can be used orally or topically.

Known properties

- anti-inflammatory, antimicrobial, antihypertensive, antipyretic, antianemic, antidiabetic, and antihemorrhagic.

Species gossypifolia means cotton-like plant, possible resembling Gossypium. Medicinal: The leaves of the plant are used for intermittent fevers, carbuncles, eczema, itches, sores on the tongues of babies, swollen mammae, stomachache, and venereal disease. The leaf decoction is used for bathing wounds.

Tea Preparation:

The leaves are used to make a tea through decoction, maceration, or infusion.

Potential Benefits:

Studies suggest that J. gossypiifolia may have anti-inflammatory, antineoplastic, antimicrobial, antioxidant, antihypertensive, and anticholinesterase activities.

How to Make Jatropha Gossypiifolia Tea (Traditional Use)

Ingredients:

- 1 small fresh leaf (or about 1 tsp chopped)
- 1–2 cups water
- Optional: ginger, lemongrass, or other herbs to reduce bitterness

Yarrow

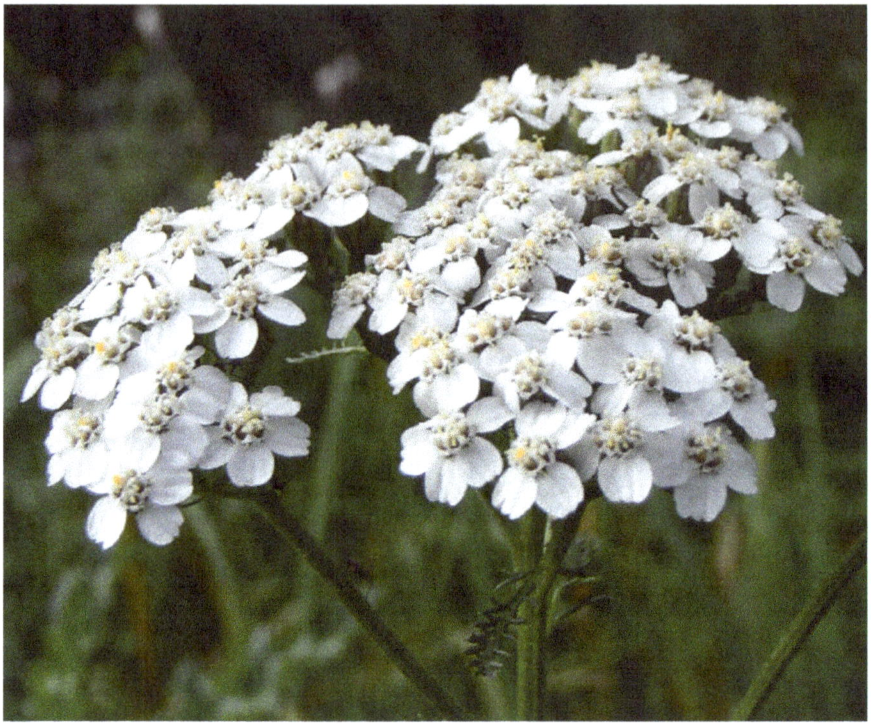

Yarrow tea may have some health benefits, including reduced inflammation, improved digestive health, and wound healing.

Yarrow tea is brewed from a popular medicinal herb.
Yarrow (Achillea millefolium) has been used for thousands of years for its potential health benefits. Its genus name, Achillea, refers to the warrior Achilles in Greek mythology, as he used yarrow to treat his soldiers' wounds.

There are 140 different species of Achillea, which are characterized by their clustered flowers and hairy, aromatic leaves.
Some research indicates this plant may have various benefits, including helping withTrusted Source inflammation, wound healing, and digestive health.

Digestive issues

Yarrow has long been used to treat digestive issues like ulcers and irritable bowel syndrome (IBS), symptoms of which include stomach pain, diarrhea, bloating, and constipation. This research found that the aerial parts of these plants (the parts above the soil) may contain a bitter digestive tonic, which might help support bile flow and work as a diuretic. The alkaloids in the plant's levels may also have antioxidant and gastroprotective properties, to help with your overall digestive health.

Symptoms of depression and anxiety

The flavonoids and alkaloids in yarrow tea may help reduce symptoms of depression and anxiety.

Brain health

2017 research suggests that yarrow may help with certain brain disorders, including multiple sclerosis, Alzheimer's, Parkinson's, and inflammation of the brain and spinal cord caused by a viral infection.

A 2018 research review also made similar findings, noting that the alkaloids present in yarrow may offer possible help for several neurodegenerative diseases, as well as possibly for stroke.

Inflammation

While inflammation is a natural bodily response, chronic inflammation can lead to cell, tissue, and organ damage.

Research indicates that yarrow has anti-inflammatory effects. Some have used yarrow and yarrow tea to help with symptoms related to inflammation. This may also include possibly reducing skin and liver inflammation and treating skin infections, aging skin, and non-alcoholic fatty liver disease.

Following the COVID-19 pandemic, this 2023 research also noted that the anti-inflammatory effects of yarrow could also help with the virus causing COVID-19.

Making yarrow tea is a soothing way to enjoy the health benefits of this ancient herb. Yarrow (Achillea millefolium) is traditionally used for fever, digestion, cramps, colds, and inflammation. It has a slightly bitter, earthy taste—so it's often blended with other herbs like mint or chamomile.

How to Make Yarrow Tea

Ingredients:

- 1–2 teaspoons dried yarrow (leaves and flowers)
- or 1 tablespoon of fresh yarrow
- 1 cup boiling water
- Optional: honey, lemon, mint, or chamomile for flavor

Steps:

1. Add the yarrow to a cup, mug, or teapot.
2. Pour 1 cup of boiling water over the herb.
3. Cover and let it steep for 10–15 minutes.
4. Strain out the herbs.
5. Add honey or lemon if the taste is too bitter.
6. Sip warm — best enjoyed when you're feeling under the weather or before bed.

Cactus

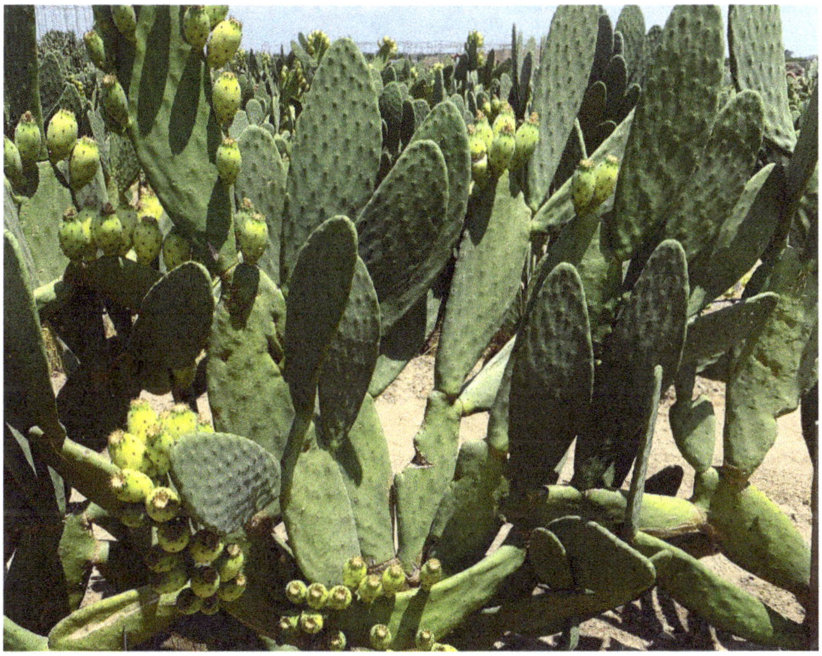

Cactus can be nutritious and may have several health benefits, including reducing inflammation, lowering blood sugar, and improving digestion.

Nutrition

- Fiber: High in fiber, which can help lower cholesterol
- Vitamins and minerals: Contains vitamins A, C, and K, as well as calcium, magnesium, potassium, and iron
- Antioxidants: Contains flavonoids and carotenoids, which have anti-inflammatory properties
- Omega-3s: Contains "good" fats
- Water: Cactus pads are about 85% water
- Potential health benefits
- Lower blood sugar
- Some research shows that people who eat cactus pads regularly have lower blood sugar

- The potassium in cactus helps your body absorb nutrients, and betalains help protect your digestive tract

- Reduce inflammation

- Cactus contains flavonoids and betalains, which have anti-inflammatory properties

Reduce the effects of a hangover

Prickly pear juice can reduce nausea, dry mouth, and other symptoms of a hangover

Edible parts

You can eat the leaves, flowers, stems, and fruit of the prickly pear cactus. You can boil or grill it, or make it into juice or jam.

How to Eat Nopales (Cactus Pads)

Cleaning & Prep:

- Use gloves or tongs — those tiny thorns (glochids) can get ya!
- Rinse the pad under water.
- Using a sharp knife, scrape off all the spines and edges.
- Wash again to make sure it's clean.
- Cut into thin strips or small cubes.

Cooking Methods:

Boiled:

- Boil chopped nopales in water with a bit of salt for 10–15 minutes.
- Drain and rinse to reduce the slimy texture (like okra).
- Grilled/Sautéed:
- Toss with a little oil, garlic, onion, and sauté until tender.
- Grill whole pads until slightly charred and soft, then slice
- Taste: Slightly tangy and crunchy, kinda like green beans meets bell pepper.

Borage

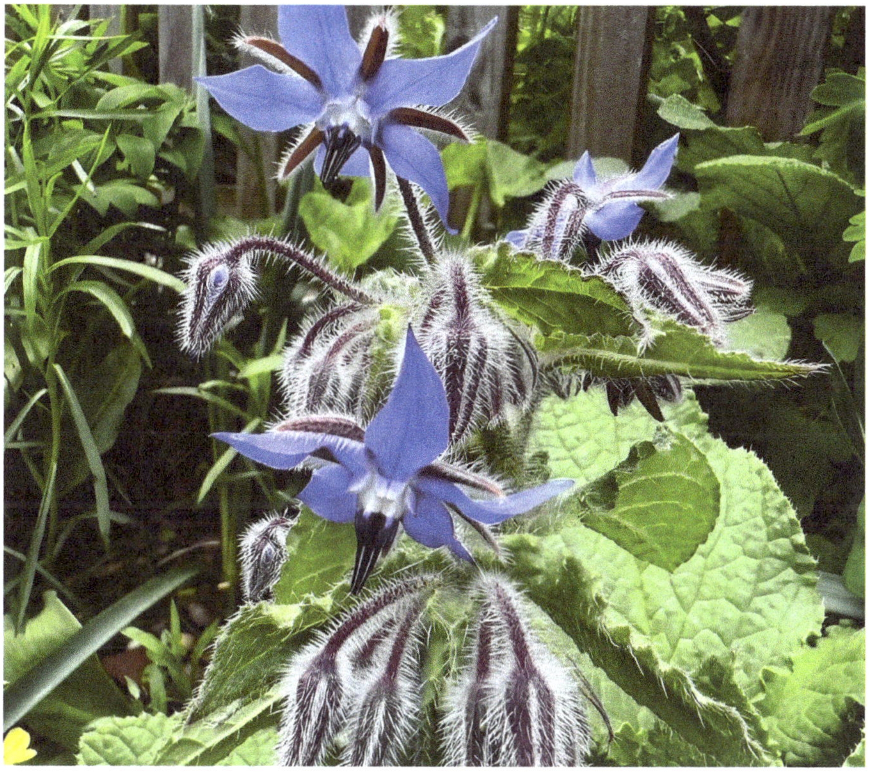

Borage is an herb that has long been prized for its health-promoting properties. It's especially rich in gamma linoleic acid (GLA), which is an omega-6 fatty acid that has been shown to decrease inflammation.
Borage may also help treat several conditions, including asthma, rheumatoid arthritis, and atopic dermatitis

What is borage?
Also known as starflower, borage is an herb notable for its vibrant purple flowers and medicinal properties.In traditional medicine, borage has been used to dilate blood vessels, act as a sedative, and treat seizures.

Both the leaves and flowers of the plant are edible and commonly used as a garnish, dried herb, or vegetable in a variety of drinks and dishes.The leaves are sometimes also ground up and steeped in hot water to brew herbal tea.

Meanwhile, the seeds are used to make borage oil, which is usually applied topically to the hair and skin. Furthermore, borage is widely available in supplement form and used to treat a variety of respiratory and digestive disorders.

May help treat asthma

Several studies have found that borage extract could help relieve symptoms of asthma by decreasing inflammation and swelling in the airways.

In one study, consuming capsules containing borage oil and echium seed oil daily for 3 weeks decreased levels of inflammation in 37 people with mild asthma.

Another 12-week study in 43 children found that taking a supplement containing borage oil, along with a blend of other ingredients like fish oil, vitamins, and minerals, decreased inflammation and symptoms of asthma

May promote skin health

Borage oil contains high amounts of gamma linolenic acid (GLA), a fatty acid that's integral to the structure and function of your skin.

Borage oil also boasts anti-inflammatory and antioxidant properties, which can help promote wound healing and repair your skin's natural barrier.

Some research has found that borage may benefit several common skin conditions, including atopic dermatitis, which is a type of eczema.

In one study, wearing an undershirt coated in borage oil every day for 2 weeks significantly improved redness and itching in 32 children with atopic dermatitis

You can also find softgel supplements at many health stores and pharmacies, typically in doses ranging from 300–1,000 mg.

Loose-leaf or prepackaged teas are available as well, which can be steeped in hot water to make a soothing cup of borage tea.

How to Make Borage Tea

Ingredients:

- 1–2 teaspoons fresh borage leaves or flowers
- (or 1 teaspoon dried leaves/flowers)
- 1 cup boiling water
- Optional: honey, lemon, or mint

Asian Ginseng

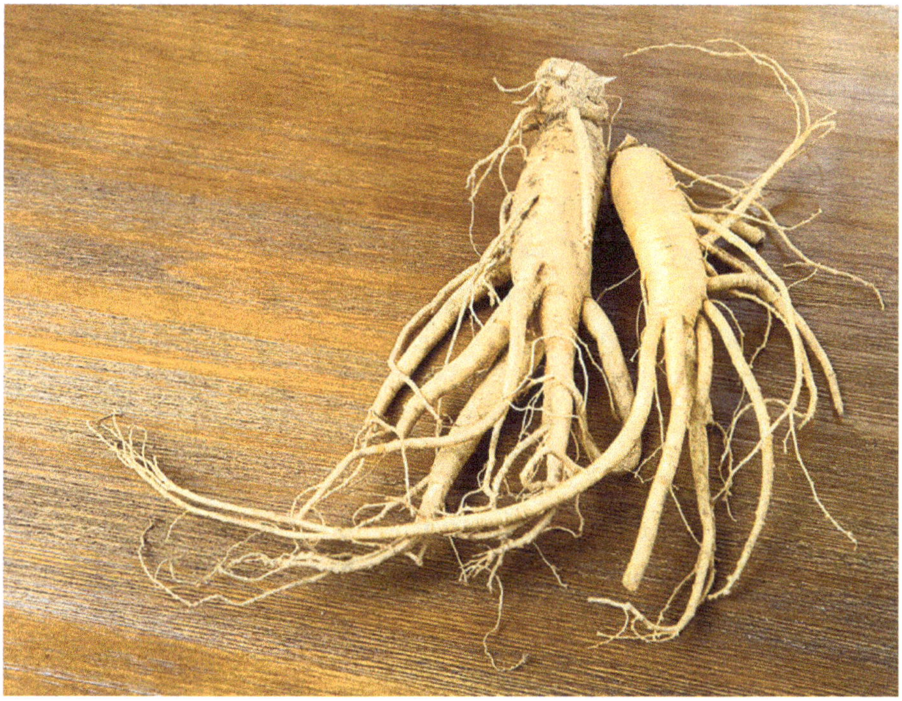

Ginseng is an herb rich in antioxidants. It may offer benefits for brain health, immune function, blood sugar management, and more. However, more research is necessary.

Ginseng has been used in traditional Chinese medicine (TCM) for centuries. It's a slow-growing short plant with fleshy roots that, depending on how long it's grown, can be classified as fresh, white, or red.

There are many varieties of this herb, including American ginseng (Panax quinquefolius) and Asian ginseng (Panax ginseng).
American and Asian ginseng vary in their concentration of active compounds and effects on the body.

Ginseng contains two significant compounds: ginsenosides and gintonin. These compounds complement one another to provide possible health benefits.

May benefit brain function

Ginseng could help improve brain functions like memory, behavior, and mood.
A 2018 study of 6,422 older adults found that regular consumption of ginseng for at least 5 years was associated with improved cognitive function later in life.

According to a 2017 study, ginseng could also help ease stress and may offer benefits for depression and anxiety.

A small 2015 study showed that taking 200 milligrams (mg) of American ginseng significantly improved working memory after 3 hours compared with a placebo.

A 2018 review explains that ginseng can have a positive effect on brain function in people with Alzheimer's disease.

Could improve erectile dysfunction

A 2021 study suggests that ginseng may be a useful alternative for the treatment of erectile dysfunction (ED). A 2022 study shows that ginseng may promote the production of nitric oxide, a compound that improves muscle relaxation in the penis and increases blood circulation. A 2021 review suggests that nitric oxide may play a role in erectile dysfunction.

May boost the immune system

According to a 2020 review, ginseng possesses potent antibacterial, antifungal, and antiviral properties. It may enhance the function of the immune system.

Interestingly, a 2018 animal study found that black red ginseng extract (BRGE) increased the number of immune cells and enhanced antioxidant levels in the liver.

Similarly, a 2020 study of 100 people showed that taking 2 grams (g) of Korean red ginseng per day for 8 weeks significantly increased levels of immune cells compared with a placebo.

How to Make Ginseng Tea (with Root)

Ingredients:

- 1–2 teaspoons of sliced ginseng root (fresh or dried)
- 1–2 cups water
- Optional: honey, lemon, ginger (for flavor)

Instructions:

1. Rinse the root under cool water.
2. Place it in a small pot with the water.
3. Bring to a boil, then reduce to a simmer.
4. Simmer gently for 10–20 minutes (longer = stronger tea).
5. Strain into a cup.
6. Add honey or lemon if desired

Maca

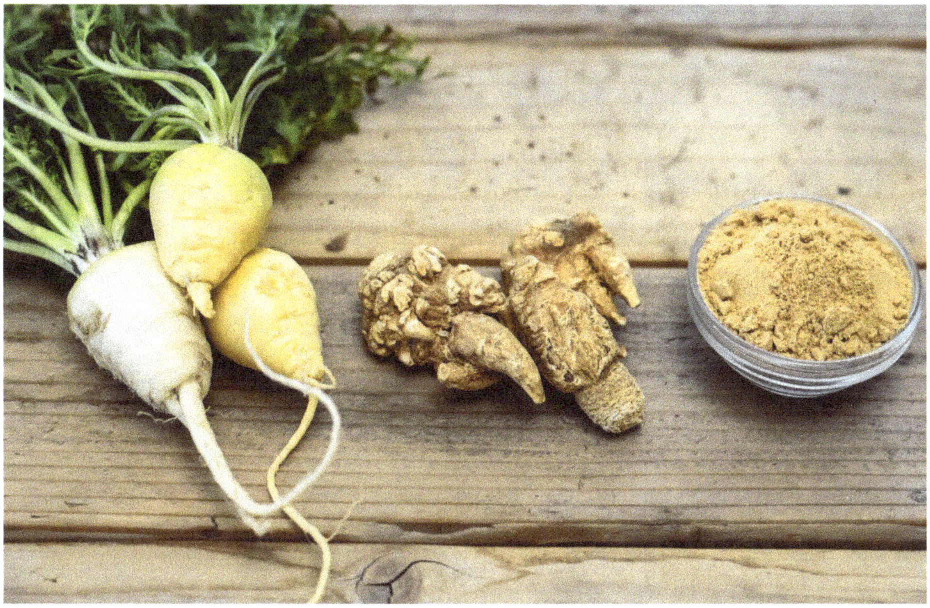

Although research on the potential health effects of maca is limited, some evidence suggests maca supplements may help improve certain aspects of sexual health and fertility, reduce menopause symptoms, and improve mood in certain people

Maca is a Peruvian plant that may have various health benefits, such as boosting libido, increasing fertility, boosting energy, and improving mood. It may also help manage menopause symptoms and blood pressure.
Maca grows in the Andes mountains. It is a cruciferous vegetable, meaning that it is related to broccoli, cabbage, and kale.

Maca is a common ingredient in Peruvian cooking that gives dishes an earthy flavor. People can grind the maca root plant into a powder and add it to meals or smoothies. Aside from its culinary uses, maca may also have several health benefits.

The most well-known benefit of maca root is its potential to increase libido. There is some scientific evidence to support this claim.
Online vendors widely promote the ability of maca root to increase libido, and this finding comes from health research.

Reducing erectile dysfunction

Maca root could also have benefits for people with erectile dysfunction (ED).
A 2023 trial found that the consumption of gelatinized maca root helped reduce ED in people with late onset hypogonadism. However, more research is necessary to fully confirm these findings.

Fighting free radicals

Maca root may also promote the production of antioxidant enzymes in the body, such as glutathione peroxidase and superoxide dismutase.
Antioxidants help fight off free radicals, which can damage cells in the body. Some research suggests antioxidants can help prevent some health conditions, including heart disease and cancer.

How to Use Maca Powder

1. Smoothies

- Blend 1–2 teaspoons of maca powder into your morning smoothie. It pairs well with bananas, cacao, peanut butter, or almond milk.

2. Tea / Hot Drinks

- Stir maca into warm (not boiling) water, or mix it into coffee, matcha, or golden milk. It has a malty, earthy flavor.

3. Oatmeal or Porridge

- Mix it in after cooking. A teaspoon or two gives your breakfast a nutrition boost.

4. Baking

- You can add maca to muffins, pancakes, or energy balls. Heat may reduce some benefits, but it still adds flavor and minerals.

5. Yogurt or Cereal

- Just sprinkle and stir.

Barrenwort/Epimedium Genus

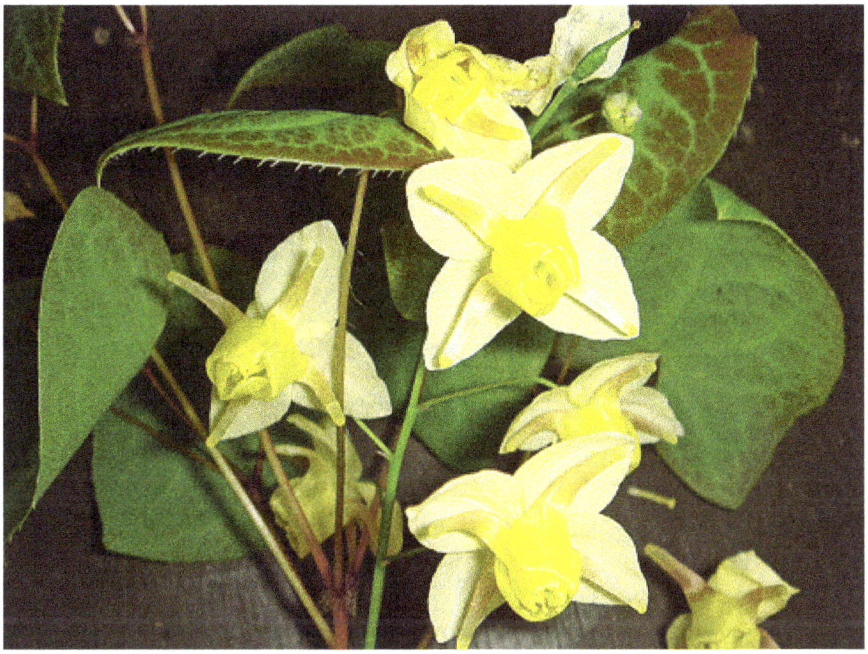

Epimedium, the suspected active component of horny goat weed, appears to increase blood flow and improve sexual function, or act as a phosphodiesterase inhibitor, similar to some drugs used for ED. Horny goat weed also contains phytoestrogens, chemicals that act somewhat like the hormone estrogen.

Its use lowers blood sugar levels. It is used in the treatment of impotence, seminal emissions, lumbago, arthritis, numbness and weakness of the limbs, hypertension and chronic bronchitis

Studies have shown that Epimedium possesses multispectral therapeutic activities, including slow aging, preventing osteoporosis, boosting immunity, anti-depression, anti-myocardial ischemia, treating erectile dysfunction, and antineoplastic effects

Barrenwort, also known as Epimedium, is most commonly used as a herbal supplement in the form of capsules, tablets, or liquid extracts, typically taken orally to potentially support sexual health, energy levels, and bone density; it can also be grown as an ornamental plant in gardens due to its attractive foliage and flowers, requiring minimal maintenance and thriving in shady areas with well-drained soil.

How to use barrenwort as a supplement:

Dosage:

Follow the recommended dosage on the product label, which usually varies depending on the form and concentration of the supplement.

Form:

Barrenwort can be found as capsules, tablets, tinctures (liquid extracts), or powders, which can be mixed into drinks.

Timing:

How to Make Barrenwort (Epimedium) Tea

Ingredients:

- 1 teaspoon dried Epimedium leaves
- 1 cup hot (not boiling) water – around 90°C / 194°F
- Optional: honey or lemon (to offset the bitter taste)

Instructions:

1. Place the dried barrenwort leaves in a cup or teapot.
2. Pour the hot water over the herbs.
3. Cover and steep for 10–15 minutes.
4. Strain and drink warm.
5. Sweeten with a little honey if desired — the taste is earthy and slightly bitter.

Take as directed by your healthcare provider, but generally, it is recommended to take it with meals for better absorption.

Important considerations when using barrenwort:

Consult a healthcare professional:

Before using barrenwort, especially if you have any underlying health conditions, are taking medications, or are pregnant or breastfeeding, talk to your doctor to ensure it is safe for you.

Lemon Peel

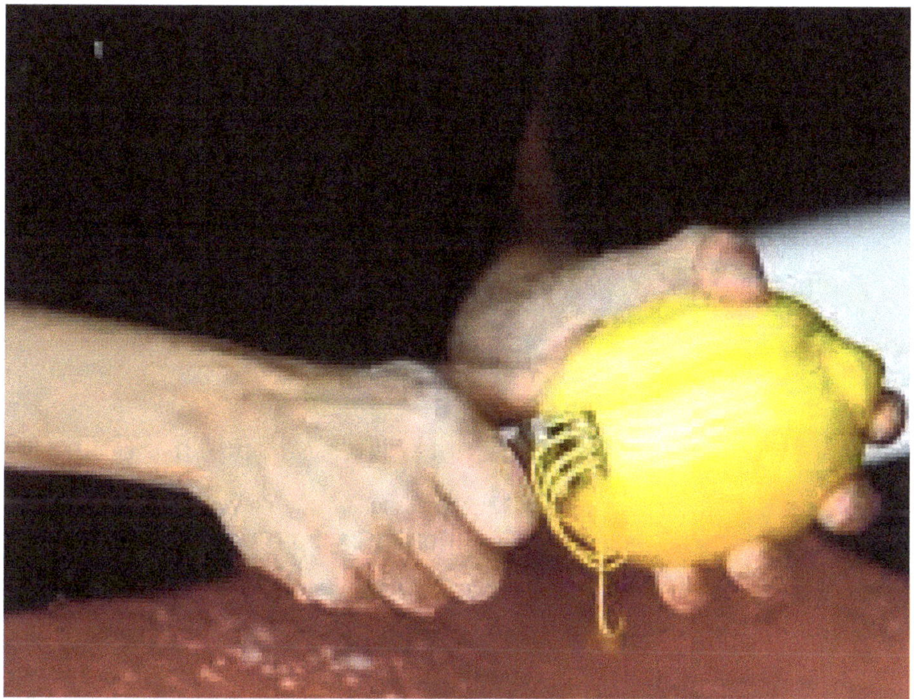

Benefits and Uses of Lemon Peel

Research shows lemon peels have many health benefits because of fiber, vitamin, and antioxidants, which can help your teeth, heart, and immune system. These fruit peels may also help fight cancer.

Lemon (Citrus limon) is a common citrus fruit, alongside grapefruits, limes, and oranges. While the pulp and juice are used the most, the peel tends to be discarded. However, studies have determined that lemon peel is full of bioactive compounds that may provide numerous health benefits.

High nutritional value

Despite being eaten in small amounts, lemon peels are very nutritious. One tablespoon (6 grams) provides:

- Calories: 3
- Carbs: 1 gram
- Fiber: 1 gram
- Protein: 0 grams
- Fat: 0 grams
- Vitamin C: 9% of the Daily Value (DV)

May support oral health

Dental cavities and gum infections are widespread oral diseases caused by bacteria like Streptococcus mutans (4Trusted Source).

Lemon peel contains antibacterial substances that may inhibit microorganism growth.

In one study, researchers identified four compounds in lemon peel that have powerful antibacterial properties and effectively fight common oral-disease-causing bacteria.

What's more, a test-tube study found that lemon peel extract combats Streptococcus mutans activity, with higher doses being more effective

High in antioxidants

Antioxidants are plant compounds that prevent cellular damage by fighting free radicals in your body.

Lemon peel is high in antioxidants, including D-limonene and vitamin C.

Intake of flavonoid antioxidants like D-limonene is linked to a reduced risk of certain conditions, such as heart disease and type 2 diabetes.

One test-tube study determined that lemon peel had stronger antioxidant activity than grapefruit or tangerine peels.

Animal studies also show that D-limonene increases the activity of an enzyme that helps reduce oxidative stress. Oxidative stress is associated with tissue damage and accelerated aging.

Additionally, the vitamin C in lemon peel acts as a powerful antioxidant and likewise promotes immune health.

Lemon Peel Tea

- Boil fresh or dried lemon peels in water for 5–10 mins.
- Add honey or ginger if you like.
- Helps with digestion and bloating.
- 4. Infused Water or Drinks
- Add lemon peels to hot water, tea, or even cocktails for a citrusy twist.

Jackass Bitters

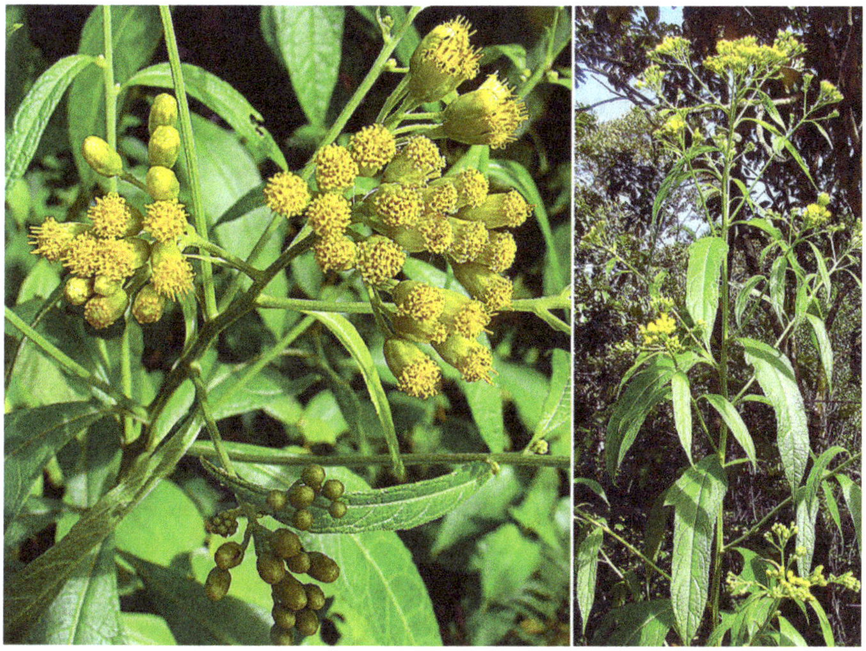

Jackass bitters, also known as Neurolaena lobata, is a plant used in traditional medicine for its potential benefits including aiding digestion, combating parasites, and potentially managing diabetes, with some research suggesting it has antimicrobial and anti-inflammatory properties.

Here's a more detailed look at the potential benefits and uses of Jackass Bitters:
Traditional Uses and Potential Benefits:

Digestive Aid:
Jackass bitters is believed to stimulate digestion by increasing saliva production and gastric juices, which may help with heartburn, cramping, and indigestion.

Anti-parasitic:
It's known for its potent anti-parasitic properties, traditionally used to treat intestinal parasites, fungal infections, and even malaria.

Diabetes Management:
Some research suggests that Jackass Bitters may help regulate blood glucose levels, potentially aiding in diabetes management.
Skin Conditions:

The plant has been used to treat skin diseases, including ringworm, and as an insect repellent.

Wound Healing:

Jackass Bitters is thought to have wound-healing properties, potentially helping to arrest bleeding, inhibit bacterial growth, and accelerate wound healing.

Other Traditional Uses:

In various regions, Jackass Bitters has been used for conditions like malaria, high blood pressure, liver problems, and as a general pain reliever.

Sesquiterpene Lactones:

The leaves contain sesquiterpene lactones, including neurolenins A, B, C, D, E, and F, and lobatin A, which are believed to be responsible for the plant's medicinal properties.

Antimicrobial and Antifungal Properties:

Research highlights the potent antimicrobial and antifungal properties of Jackass Bitters, particularly against Candida species and various bacteria.

Anti-inflammatory and Antioxidant Properties:

Some studies suggest that Jackass Bitters may possess anti-inflammatory and antioxidant properties.

Preparation Methods:

- Internal Use: Boil a handful of leaves in a liter of water and drink throughout the day.

Skin Infections:

- Mash fresh leaves and apply directly to the affected area.
- Urinary Issues: Prepare a tea using the flowers.

Peperomia pellucida

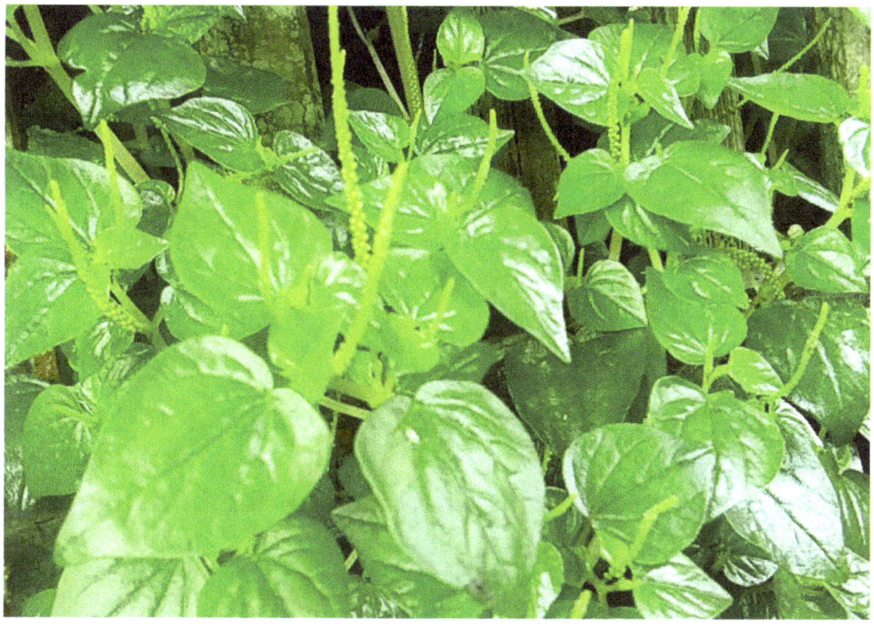

P. pellucida has been used for treating abdominal pain, abscesses, acne, boils, colic, fatigue, gout, headache, renal disorders, and rheumatic joint pain. In Bolivia, Alteños Indians use the whole plant to stop hemorrhages. The roots are used to treat fevers and the aerial parts are used as dressing for wounds

Peperomia pellucida, known as "pansit-pansitan" or "crab claw herb," is a medicinal plant used in traditional medicine for various ailments, including treating headaches, fevers, wounds, and kidney problems, and it also has potential as a source of protein and minerals.

Peperomia pellucida, a plant with traditional uses, has shown potential as an antihypertensive agent, potentially due to its ACE-inhibitory activity, which can lower blood pressure.

Edible Uses:

Salads: The leaves and shoots can be added to salads for a mild, slightly mustard-like flavor.

Cooked Greens: You can cook the leaves and stems as you would other leafy greens.

Tea: Boil the leaves to create a tea that some people find has a minty taste.

Other preparations: Some people also chew the leaves or use them as a flavoring agent in cooking.

FOR INTERNAL BLEEDING (e.g. mild ulcers, stomach lining issues, blood in urine):

- Method 2: Herbal Decoction (Mild Tea)
- Wash a handful of fresh leaves.
- Boil in 2–3 cups of water for 10–15 minutes.
- Let cool, then strain.
- Drink 1/2 cup 2–3 times a day for 2–3 days only.

Traditionally used for blood in urine, heavy menstruation, or ulcers—but not meant for long-term use without a herbalist or doctor's guidance

Leaf of Life

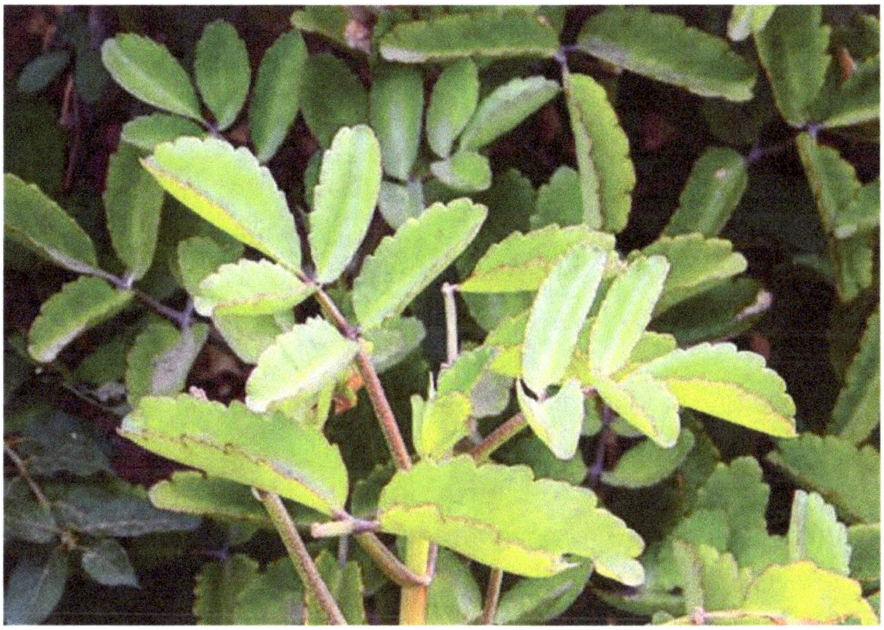

Native to Madagascar, the Leaf of Life love-bush symbolises the regenerative power of life with its green fleshy appearance. It moisturises our lives with its succulent properties.

Geological distribution

This wild herb, also known as Cathedral Bells, is found extensively in the Caribbean, Indian sub-continent, Brazil and the United States. It is a succulent perennial herb which grows up to 2 metres in height.

Each plant grows as the leaf drops into the soil emerging as a new plant.
It can adapt to water-stress like a sponge and retains water for dry times. Cathedral Bells grow from the black dot on the plant which acts as a seed.

The edges of the leaves are jagged and the flower of the plant blooms over the stem at the very top. They grow in different colours ranging from pink, red and purple to greenish and the flowers usually appear in spring and winter.
The incredible health benefits of this plant have attracted investors to grow it on a commercial scale to cater to the pharmaceutical and cosmetic industry.

Herbal tea from the Leaf of Life plant leaves has cured shortness of breath, coughs and colds.
Tea infused with the leaves acts as a diuretic and helps reduce high blood pressure, though mildly sedative in nature.
The crushed leaves are mixed with coconut oil and are used for curing headaches.

How to Make Leaf of Life Tea

You'll Need:

- 2–3 fresh Leaf of Life leaves
- 2 cups water
- Optional: ginger, honey, or lime for extra taste and benefits

Instructions:

1. Wash the leaves thoroughly to remove any dirt or residue.
2. Tear or cut them into smaller pieces (no need to remove the skin).
3. Bring 2 cups of water to a boil.
4. Add the leaves and simmer on low heat for 5–10 minutes.
5. Turn off heat and let it steep for another 5 minutes.
6. Strain, then sweeten with honey or add lime juice if desired.
7. Drink warm, preferably once or twice a day when treating symptoms.

Common Uses of Leaf of Life Tea:

- Clears chest congestion and mucus
- Helps soothe asthma, coughs, and bronchitis
- Reduces fever
- Supports urinary health and detox
- Promotes wound healing and immune support

Caution

It is used widely for skin hydration.
The plant should not be consumed during pregnancy.

Pigeon Peas Leaves

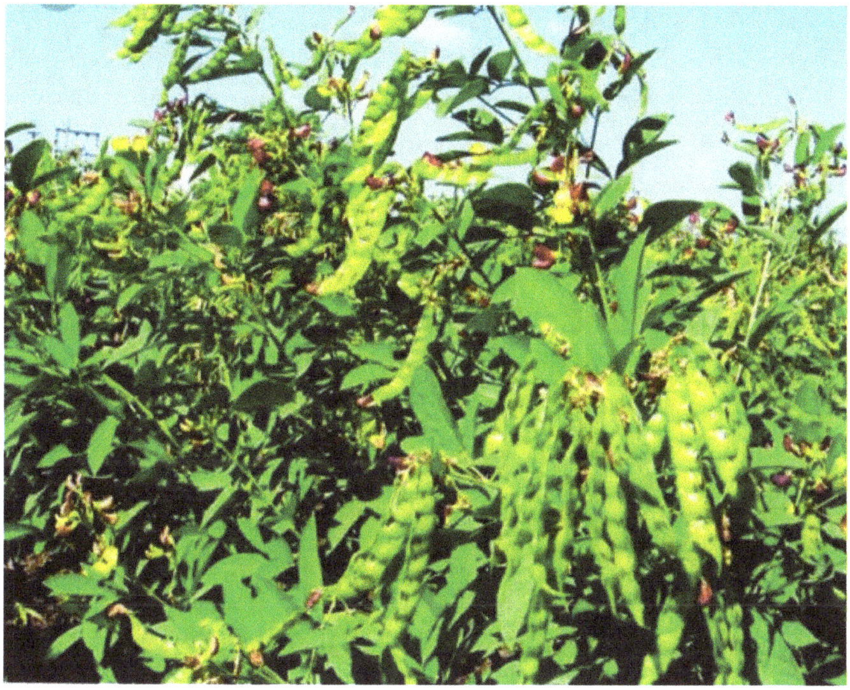

Pigeon pea leaves, rich in bioactive compounds like phenolic compounds and flavonoids, offer potential health benefits including anti-inflammatory, antibacterial, antioxidant, and antidiabetic effects.

Here's a more detailed look at the potential benefits:
Rich in Bioactive Compounds: Pigeon pea leaves contain various beneficial compounds, including phenolic compounds, flavonoids, tannins, saponins, and phytic acid.

Anti-inflammatory Properties: These compounds contribute to the plant's anti-inflammatory properties.
Antibacterial Activity: Pigeon pea leaves have demonstrated antibacterial activity.
Antioxidant Effects: The presence of antioxidants helps protect against cellular damage.

Antidiabetic Potential: Pigeon pea has been linked to antidiabetic effects.
Other potential benefits: Pigeon pea leaves have been traditionally used to treat various conditions, including fever, dysentery, and jaundice.
Nutritional value: Pigeon pea leaves are also a good source of carbohydrates, starch, and dietary fiber.

Pigeon pea leaf tea, made from the leaves of the Cajanus cajan plant, is believed to offer various health benefits, including potential anti-inflammatory, antibacterial, and antioxidant properties, as well as being used in traditional medicine for conditions like fever and dysentery.

Here's a more detailed look at the potential benefits:
Traditional Uses:

Pigeon pea leaves have been used in traditional medicine for treating conditions like fever, dysentery, and to kill parasites.
In some parts of Tamil Nadu, India, the leaves, seeds, and young stems are used to cure gingivitis, stomatitis, and as a toothbrush.
Pigeon pea leaves are also believed to cure typhoid.

How to Make Pigeon Leaf Tea

You'll Need:

- A handful of fresh pigeon pea leaves (or 1–2 teaspoons dried leaves)
- 2 cups water
- Optional: ginger, honey, garlic, lime

Instructions:

1. Wash the leaves thoroughly.
2. Add them to 2 cups of boiling water.
3. Lower heat and simmer for 10–15 minutes.
4. Turn off heat, cover, and let steep another 5 minutes.
5. Strain and serve warm.
6. Add honey or lime juice if you like

Chinkweed

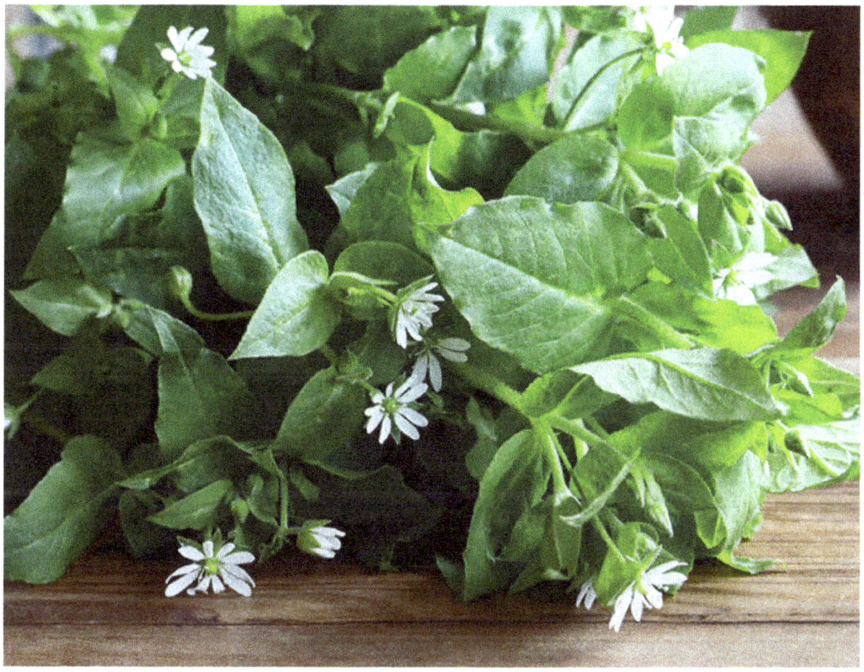

Chickweed, a common herb, is traditionally used for its cooling and anti-inflammatory properties, potentially aiding in wound healing, soothing skin irritations, and supporting digestive health.

Here's a more detailed look at the potential benefits and uses of chickweed:

Traditional and Potential Uses:

Skin Soothing:

- Chickweed is known for its ability to soothe irritated skin, making it a popular choice for treating conditions like eczema, psoriasis, and rashes.

Wound Healing:

- Chickweed is believed to promote wound healing and may help fight germs and infections.

Anti-inflammatory Properties:

- Chickweed contains compounds like saponins and flavonoids, which are known for their anti-inflammatory effects.

Digestive Support:

- Chickweed has been traditionally used as a digestive tonic, potentially supporting healthy bowel movements and soothing inflammation in the gastrointestinal tract.

Other Traditional Uses:

Chickweed has been used as a folk remedy for various conditions, including asthma, blood disorders, conjunctivitis, constipation, inflammation, dyspepsia, skin ailments, and obesity.

Edible Plant:

The young shoots of chickweed are edible and can be consumed raw as a salad green or cooked like spinach.

While some anecdotal evidence suggests chickweed tea might help shrink fibroids.

How Chinkweed Helps with Fibroids

- **Anti-inflammatory**: May reduce swelling and pain caused by fibroids
- **Hormone balancing:** Traditionally believed to help regulate estrogen levels
- **Uterine tonic**: Used to tone and cleanse the womb
- **Blood purifier:** Supports overall detoxification

How to Make Chinkweed Tea

You'll Need:

- 1 handful of fresh chinkweed leaves (or 1–2 teaspoons dried)
- 2 cups water
- Optional: ginger, turmeric, or lemon (for added benefits and taste)

Instructions:

1. Wash the leaves thoroughly.
2. Add to a pot with 2 cups of water.
3. Bring to a boil, then simmer for 10–15 minutes.
4. Remove from heat and let it steep for 5–10 more minutes.
5. Strain, and sweeten with honey or lemon juice if desired.
6. Drink 1 cup in the morning and 1 cup at night for a few days at a time.

Neem

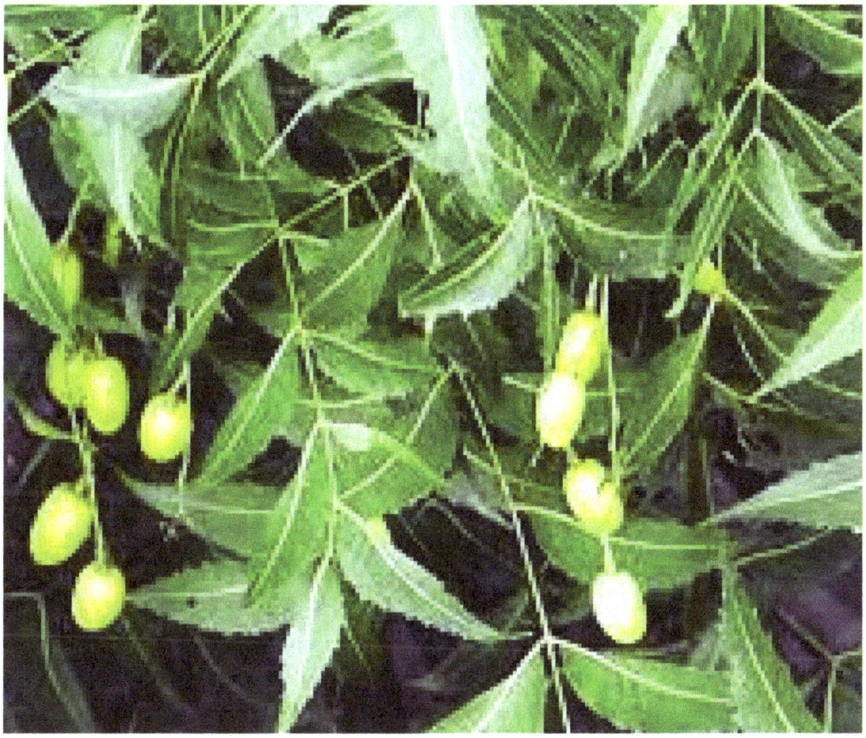

Neem offers several skin benefits due to its antimicrobial, anti-inflammatory, and antioxidant properties, including helping treat acne, soothe irritated skin, and potentially reduce signs of aging.
Here's a more detailed look at the benefits:

Acne and Blemish Treatment:
Neem's antibacterial properties can help fight acne-causing bacteria and reduce inflammation, potentially leading to clearer skin.

Soothing Irritated Skin:
Neem can soothe redness, itchiness, and inflammation, making it beneficial for conditions like eczema or psoriasis.

Moisturizing and Hydrating:
Neem oil contains fatty acids and vitamin E, which can help moisturize and hydrate dry skin, preventing flakiness and promoting a healthy skin barrier.

Reducing Signs of Aging:
Neem's antioxidants may help combat free radicals, potentially reducing the appearance of wrinkles, fine lines, and dark spots.

Promoting Wound Healing:

Neem's antimicrobial properties can help prevent infection and promote faster healing of minor wounds and cuts.

Skin Purifying:

Neem can help cleanse the skin, reduce excess oil, and tighten pores, contributing to a smoother, more even-toned complexion.

Protecting Against Environmental Damage:

Neem's antioxidant capabilities can help protect the skin from damage caused by UV radiation, pollution, and other environmental stressors.

Minimizing scars and spots

Neem can help in minimizing scars, discolouration, and spots on the face

For Skin and Hair:

Neem Oil:

- **Dilution**: Neem oil is potent and needs to be diluted before use. For skin, mix a few drops of neem oil with a carrier oil like coconut or olive oil.

- **Application:** Apply diluted neem oil to targeted areas like acne, scars, or insect bites.

- **Face Packs**: Create a face pack by mixing neem powder with ingredients like turmeric, yogurt, or rose water for acne treatment and skin soothing.

- **Moisturizing**: Neem leaves or powder can be used to moisturize the skin and treat dryness.

- **Toner**: Neem leaves can also be used as a toner to rejuvenate the skin.

Neem Leaves:

- **Paste:** Grind fresh neem leaves into a paste and apply it directly to pimples or areas of concern.

Neem Juice:

Consumption: Mix neem juice with water and consume it on an empty stomach in the morning for digestive benefits.

Skin Benefits: Neem juice can also be applied to the skin for its anti-inflammatory and antibacterial properties.

For Overall Health:

- **Drinking Neem Juice:** Neem juice can help improve digestion, enhance metabolism, and purge the colon.
- **Neem Powder**: Neem powder can be added to soups, stews, or smoothies for added nutritional value.
- **Chewing Neem Twigs**: Chewing on neem twigs can promote oral hygiene and freshen breath.
- **Neem Capsules**: Neem capsules are available as a convenient way to consume neem extracts.

How to Make Neem Juice (from Fresh Leaves)

Ingredients:

- 10–15 fresh neem leaves
- 1 cup water (cold or room temperature)
- Optional: honey, lemon, or a few mint leaves for taste

Instructions:

1. Wash the neem leaves thoroughly.
2. Add them to a blender with 1 cup of water.
3. Blend until you get a smooth, green liquid.
4. Strain the juice using a fine mesh strainer or cheesecloth.
5. Pour into a glass and add lemon juice or honey (to cut the bitterness, if needed).
6. Drink on an empty stomach in the morning, 2–3 times per week.

Horsetail

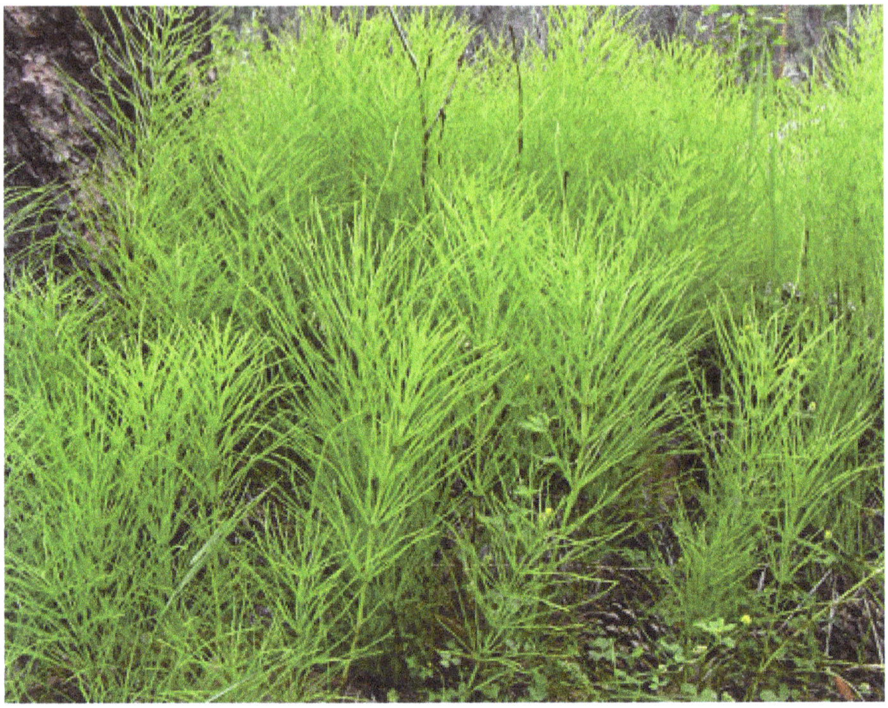

Horsetail contains silicon, which helps strengthen bone. For that reason, some practitioners recommend horsetail as a treatment for osteoporosis. It is also used as a diuretic, and as an ingredient in some cosmetics. However, few studies have investigated horsetail's effect in humans

Horsetail (Equisetum arvense) is a plant that has been used as an herbal remedy for centuries. Historically, it was used as a diuretic to increase the frequency of urination. In recent years, it has developed a reputation as a hair care and hair loss remedy.
Keep reading to learn what properties in horsetail extract may make it beneficial for your hair.

Why is horsetail used for hair?
Although the evidence is primarily anecdotal, some scientific studies indicate horsetail may promote healthy hair based on its:

- silicon content
- impact on collagen
- antioxidant properties

Silicon

Some proponents of natural remedies suggest that the silica in horsetail extract makes it a good hair care product. They back up their claims with:

- A 2016 study indicating daily doses of silicon over a 9-month period showed positive results for hair properties, such as resistance to breaking

- A 2015 study concluding oral tablets, including horsetail for natural silica, improved hair strength and growth

It's also claimed that the silicon:

- gives horsetail a texture that is useful for cleaning
- improves hair growth speed
- reduces dandruff
- boosts scalp circulation
- Collagen

Many advocates of using horsetail for hair care suggest its impact on collagen and calcium for bone regeneration are also beneficial for hair health and appearance

1. Horsetail Tea:

- **Preparation**: Steep 2-3 teaspoons of dried horsetail herb in 1 cup of boiling water for 5-10 minutes.
- **Usage**: Drink the tea 2-3 times daily.
- **External Use**: Horsetail tea can be used as a rinse for hair or as a skin tonic.

2. Horsetail Supplements:

Forms: Available as capsules, tinctures, and extracts.

- **Dosage**: Follow the instructions on the product label or consult with a healthcare professional.
- **Example**: Some supplements contain 900 mg of horsetail extract.

3. Topical Applications:

- **Skin:** Horsetail can be used as a skin tonic or in compresses.
- **Hair**: Some people use horsetail extracts in shampoos or rinses to promote hair health.
- **Wound Healing:** Horsetail has been used topically to promote wound healing.

Jack in the Bush

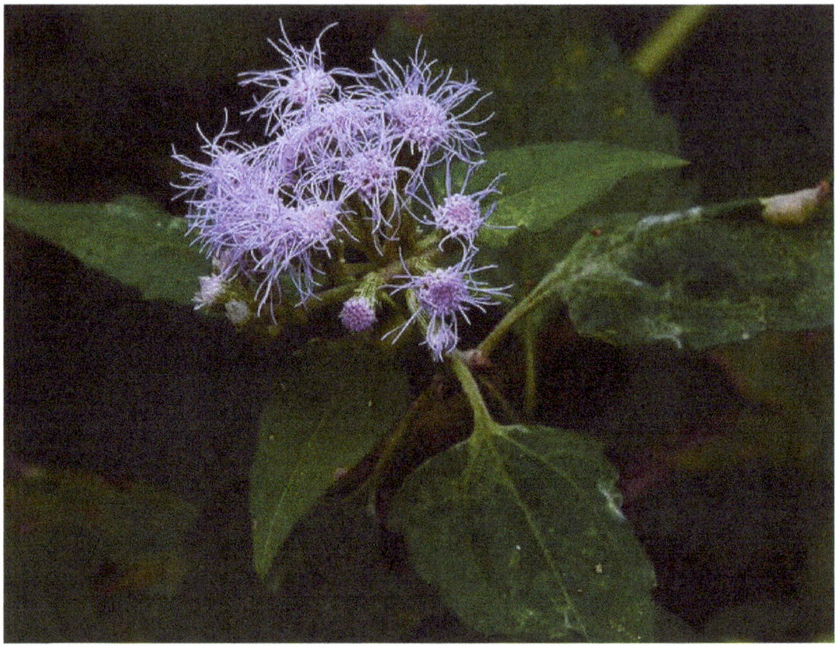

Jack in the Bush

The medicinal wonder plant, scientifically known as Eupatorium Odoratum, grow wild all over Jamaica and other parts of the Caribbean. It is also known as Christmas bush, siam weed, bitter bush and agrimony depending on the island.

Jack in the Bush reportedly contains Alpha-pinene properties that help to eliminate infections and promote healing. A tea made from the leaves is said to be excellent for flu, coughs, common colds, asthma, sinusitis as well as fever.
Persons who suffer from diabetes also reportedly stand to benefit from the tea made from the flower of the Jack in the Bush.

It is also said to be good for inflammation and to treat skin conditions such as eczema. The tea has also been used to ease the effects of measles and chicken pox.
What's more, a mixture of the shoots of the plant and coconut milk is used to help treat children who suffer from bronchitis.

How to Use Jack In The Bush?

The leaf of the Jack'na Bush is the part of the shrub that is traditionally used in herbal medicine. The leaves can be crushed in the hands or grinded before being applied to cuts on the skin.

One can then bandage the crushed leaves around that specific area of the body to promote healing. Some also inhale the pungent, aromatic odour from the crushed leaf to bring relief from coughs. The leaf of the Jack In The Bush can also be boiled with milk, or used as an ingredient to make a herbal tea, and is used to treat bronchitis and asthma along with the cold and the flu.

Jack in the Bush tea is made from the plant Eupatorium odoratum, also known in Jamaica and the Caribbean as Jack-in-the-Bush, Christmas bush, or bitter bush. It's a strong traditional bush medicine used for cleansing the womb, fever, colds, infections, and even diabetes and high blood pressure in folk remedies.

How to Make Jack-in-the-Bush Tea

You'll Need:

- 3–5 fresh Jack-in-the-Bush leaves (or 1–2 tsp dried)
- 2 cups water
- Optional: garlic, ginger, or lime for extra benefits

Instructions:

1. Wash the leaves well.
2. Bring 2 cups of water to a boil.
3. Add the leaves and simmer for 10–15 minutes.
4. Let steep another 5 minutes off the fire.
5. Strain and drink warm.
6. Sweeten with honey if desired, or drink as-is for maximum potency.

Traditional Uses:

- Cleanses the womb after childbirth or menstruation

- Used to relieve fever, cold, or flu symptoms

- Helps reduce blood sugar and blood pressure

- Acts as a diuretic and supports kidney function

- Can help with infections, especially urinary tract or internal inflammation

Hoslundia opposita

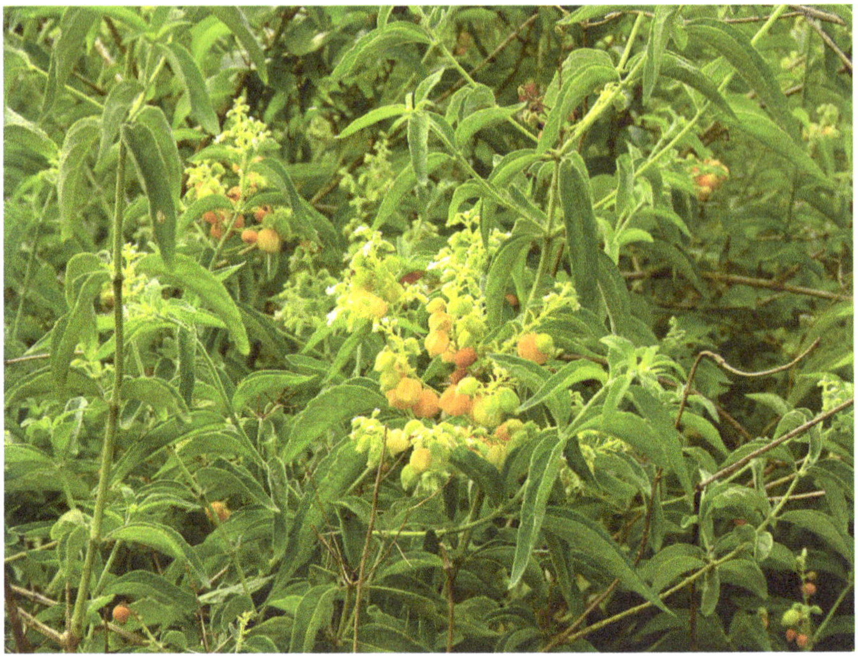

In traditional African medicine, a decoction of Hoslundia opposita (leaves and roots) is used to treat stomach ulcers, and some studies suggest its aqueous extract has anti-Helicobacter pylori and potential anti-ulcer activity.
Here's a more detailed explanation:

Traditional Use:
The plant Hoslundia opposita (also known as "Hoslundia") is a shrub used in some regions of Africa (especially sub-Saharan Africa) to treat various conditions, including chest pain, stomach pain, wounds, malaria, and sores.

Anti-ulcer Potential:
A survey by Agyare et al. showed that traditional healers used Hoslundia opposita for healing wounds and stomach ulcers.
Studies on the aqueous extract of H. opposita showed it has strong antiadhesive effects against Helicobacter pylori (a bacteria that can cause stomach ulcers), suggesting it may be useful in ulcer treatment.

Some research suggests the plant's essential oils may contribute to the treatment of stomach ulcer pain. The plant's phytochemical constituents, particularly flavonoids, are thought to have antimicrobial activity that can help prevent wound infections, which is also a factor in ulcer healing.

Here's a more detailed overview of how to use Hoslundia opposita:

Medicinal Uses:

Traditional uses in sub-Saharan Africa include treating chest pain, stomach pains, wounds, malaria, cystitis, liver diseases, epilepsy, gonorrhea, fever, cough, and sores.

Some sources mention its use for HIV/AIDS related diseases, breast cancer, appendicitis and convulsions. It may also be used post-partum to cleanse the uterus of any blood clots and heal vaginal lacerations.

Hoslundia opposita, commonly called "kamunye", is a herb used in some African regions traditionally to cleanse the uterus post-partum and heal vaginal lacerations after childbirth, often taken as a tea.

Traditional Use:

In parts of Africa, "kamunye" (Hoslundia opposita) is used traditionally post-partum to cleanse the uterus of blood clots and help heal vaginal lacerations from childbirth.

Herbal Tea:

It's commonly consumed as a tea, either alone or combined with other herbs.

Potential Benefits:

Some pharmacological investigations indicate that Hoslundia opposita might possess antimicrobial, analgesic, anti-inflammatory, and other properties.

Uses Beyond Post-partum:

Traditional healers may use Hoslundia opposita to treat wounds, stomach ulcers, and dermatitis.

How to make Hoslundia opposita tea

Ingredients:

- Fresh or dried Hoslundia opposita leaves (about a handful if fresh, or 1–2 tablespoons if dried)
- 2–3 cups of water
- (Optional) Honey or lime for taste

Willow Bark

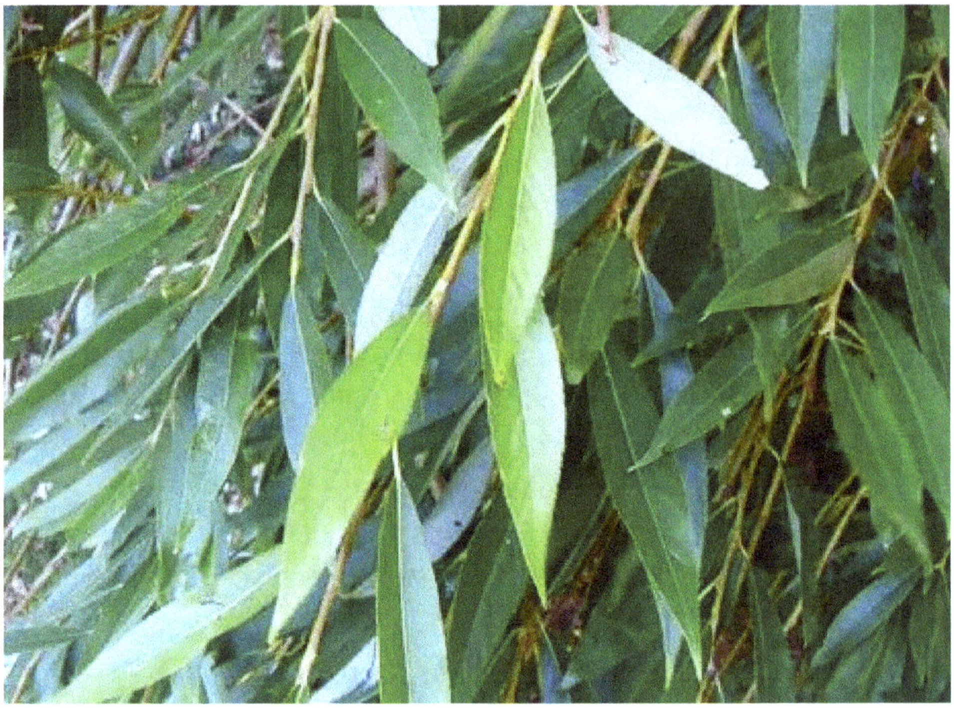

Willow bark is used to ease pain and reduce inflammation. Researchers believe that the chemical salicin, found in willow bark, is responsible for these effects.

Possibly Effective for

Back pain. Taking willow bark by mouth seems to reduce lower back pain. Higher doses seem to be more effective than lower doses, and it may take up to a week to help. There is interest in using willow bark for a number of other purposes, but there isn't enough reliable information to say whether it might be helpful.

Side Effects

When taken by mouth: Willow bark is possibly safe when used for up to 12 weeks. It might cause diarrhea, heartburn, and vomiting in some people. It can also cause itching, rash, and allergic reactions, particularly in people who are allergic to aspirin.

Special Precautions and Warnings

When taken by mouth: Willow bark is possibly safe when used for up to 12 weeks. It might cause diarrhea, heartburn, and vomiting in some people. It can also cause itching, rash, and allergic reactions, particularly in people who are allergic to aspirin.Pregnancy: There isn't enough reliable information to know if willow bark is safe to use when pregnant. Stay on the safe side and avoid use.

To make willow bark tea for pain relief, steep 1-2 teaspoons of dried white willow bark powder in 8 ounces of boiling water for 10-15 minutes, then strain and optionally sweeten with honey or add herbs like cinnamon or ginger.

Here's a more detailed breakdown:

1. Gather Your Materials:

White Willow Bark: You'll need dried white willow bark powder or small pieces of the bark.

- Water: Use clean, boiled water.
- Container: A saucepan or teapot will work well.
- Optional: Honey, cinnamon sticks, or ginger root for flavor and additional benefits.

2. Prepare the Tea:

- Boil the Water: Bring the water to a boil.
- Add Willow Bark: Place 1-2 teaspoons of dried white willow bark powder or the appropriate amount of bark chunks in the saucepan or teapot.
- Infuse: Pour the boiling water over the bark and simmer for 10-15 minutes.
- Optional Add-ins: If desired, add cinnamon sticks or sliced ginger root for flavor.
- Strain: Remove the willow bark pieces and cinnamon or ginger from the pot, leaving only the infused liquid.
- Sweeten (optional): Add honey or other sweetener to taste.

3. Drink and Enjoy (or Consider Other Uses)

Dosage: Consume 1-3 cups of the tea daily.

- **Storage:** Store any leftover tea in the refrigerator for up to 2-3 days.
- Other Uses: You can also use the steeped water as a compress for pain relief or add it to a bath.

Chanca piedra

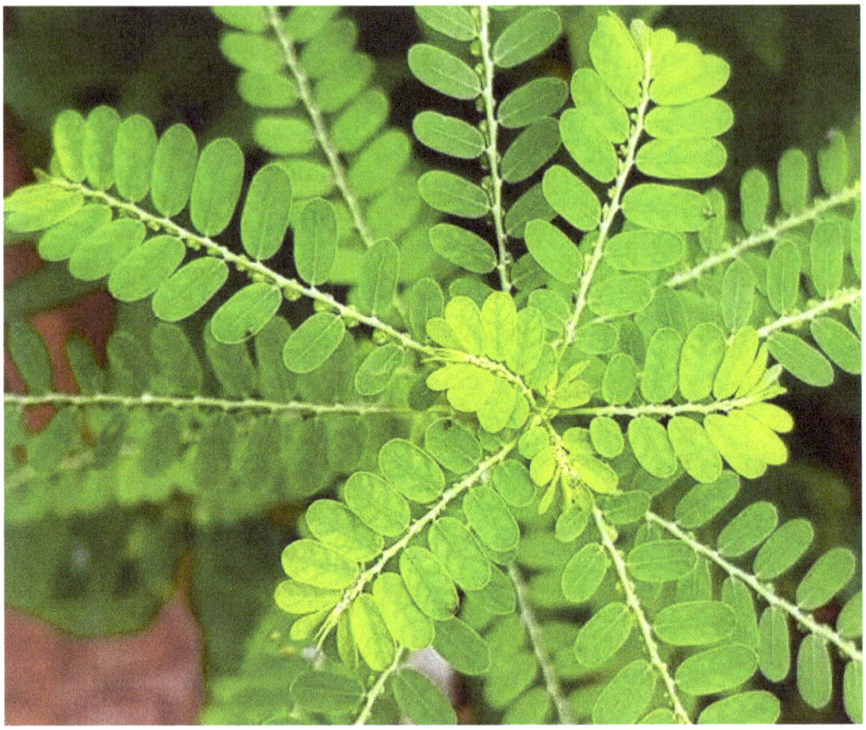

Kidney stones

Chanca piedra is best known as a potential kidney stone cure — which is how it earned the name "stone breaker."

The herb is alkaline, so it may help prevent acidic kidney stones. It's a less expensive, over-the-counter alternative to prescription potassium citrate, an alkalizing agent that's commonly used to prevent acidic kidney stones. It may also help you urinate more.

In one study of 56 people with kidney stones who took 1 cup of hot water infused with an herbal sachet containing 4.5 grams of chanca piedra twice daily, researchers found that the kidney stones decreased in size and number in about two-thirds of participants. What's more, other small human studies have observed some benefit to taking chanca piedra for kidney stones.

Gallstones

For the same reason it may help with kidney stones, the alkalizing properties of chanca piedra may help prevent gallstones as well. It's used in some traditional medicine practices as a gallstone treatment.

Gout

Gout flare-ups can occur when high levels of uric acid build up in the blood. Chanca piedra may help balance out these levels and prevent gout attacks.

Some animal studies have shown a decrease in uric acid levels in animals receiving chanca piedra supplements.

Liver disease

Due to its antioxidant content, chanca piedra may improve liver function and help protect the liver from cellular damage caused by free radicals — unstable compounds that can cause damage when they build up in your body in high levels

Chanca piedra may also reduce blood sugar and blood pressure levels, so it should be used with caution if you're on a blood pressure or blood sugar lowering medication.

Keep in mind that supplements aren't regulated by any government organizations, so there's little oversight to ensure that the label is an honest representation of what's in the supplement.

If you choose to take chanca piedra, you should buy a supplement that has been independently verified for quality by a third party organization. Some of these organizations include ConsumerLab, NSF International, and United States Pharmacopeia (USP).

Dosag

How to make chanca piedra tea

Chanca piedra tea can be consumed to prevent kidney stones made up of calcium oxalate. It can also prevent pre-existing stones from increasing in size, as this plant contains properties that prevent crystal aggregation in the urinary tract.

How to prepare

- 20 g of chance piedra
- 1 liter of water
- Boil the water and add the plant. Allow to soak for 5 to 10 minutes, then strain and drink while warm, preferably unsweetened.

Other ways this plant can be used are:

- Infusion: 20 to 30 g per liter. Consume 1 to 2 cups per day.
- Decoction: 10 a 20 g por litro. Consume 2 to 3 cups per day
- Dry extract in capsule form: 350 mg, up to 3 times per day
- Powder: 0.5 to 2 g per day
- Tincture: 10 a 20 mL, divided into 2 or 3 daily doses and diluted in a small amount of water

Cucumber Juice

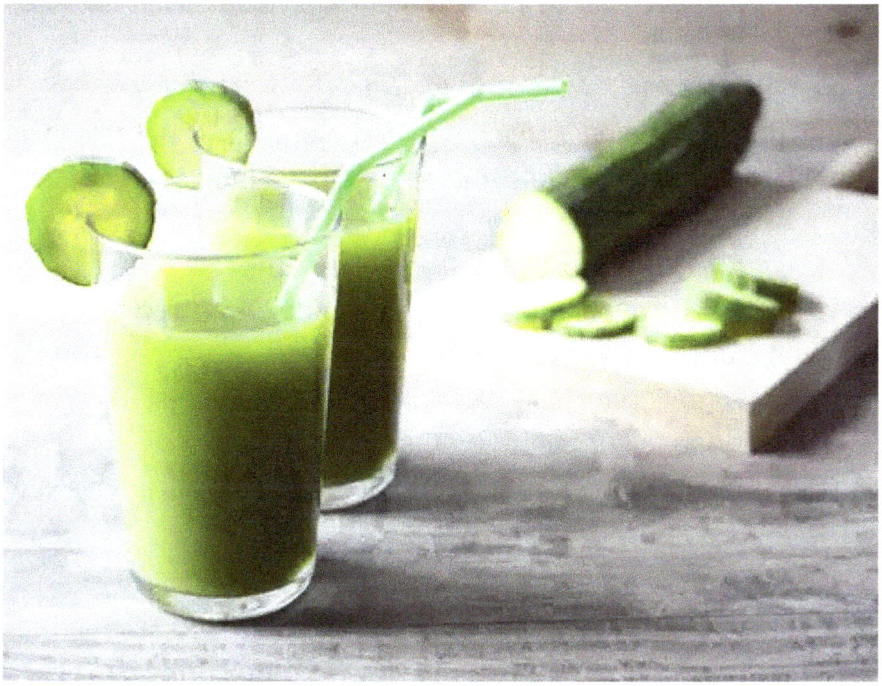

Cucumber juice can be a hydrating and potentially beneficial beverage for individuals with diabetes, offering low calories and carbohydrates, and potentially aiding in blood sugar regulation and overall health.
Here's a more detailed look at the benefits and considerations:

Potential Benefits:

Hydration:

Cucumber juice is a great source of hydration, which is crucial for overall health and can be particularly important for people with diabetes.

Low in Calories and Carbohydrates:

Cucumber juice is naturally low in calories and carbohydrates, making it a suitable beverage for individuals managing their blood sugar levels.

May Help with Blood Sugar Regulation:

Some studies suggest that cucumbers may help lower blood sugar levels and reduce the risk of hypoglycemia.

Antioxidant Rich:

Cucumbers contain antioxidants that can help protect against cell damage and reduce inflammation.

May Help Maintain Blood Pressure:

Cucumber juice can help maintain healthy blood pressure levels, which is important for overall health and can be beneficial for individuals with diabetes.

Vitamin K source:

Cucumber juice is rich in vitamin K, which can be helpful for those struggling to maintain healthy blood sugar levels and also helps in blood clotting and

How to Make Cucumber Juice:

1. Wash and chop: Wash the cucumber thoroughly and chop it into pieces.
2. Blend: Place the cucumber pieces in a blender or juicer.
3. Add other ingredients (optional): You can add other ingredients, such as lemon juice, mint, or ginger, for added flavor and nutrients.
4. Strain (optional): Strain the juice through a fine-mesh sieve to remove any pulp if desired.
5. Serve: Serve the juice chilled and enjoy.

Cucumber Juice Recipe (for Insulin Support)

Ingredients

- 1 large cucumber (organic, if possible)
- 1/2 cup water (optional, for smoother blending)
- Lime or lemon juice (optional, for flavor)
- Small piece of ginger (optional, anti-inflammatory)
- A few mint leaves (optional, refreshing)

King of the Forest

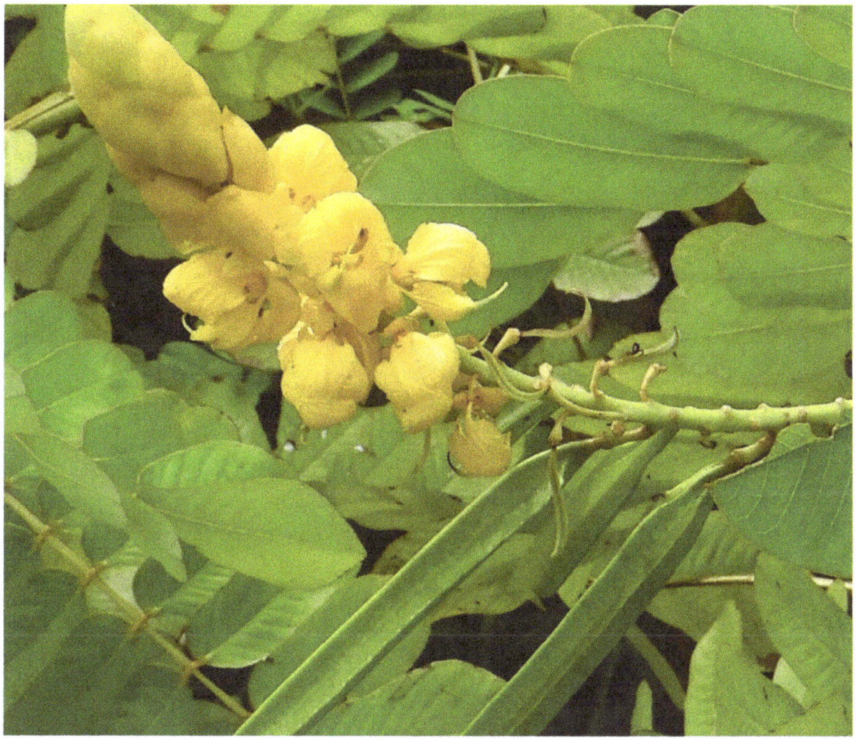

The "King of the Forest" plant, scientifically known as Senna alata or Cassia alata, is used traditionally in Jamaica and other regions for its potential medicinal benefits, including treating skin conditions, burns, and as a laxative.

Here's a more detailed look at its potential uses and properties:

Skin Conditions:

Used to treat burns, ringworm, liver spots, and fungal skin infections.

Rubbing the leaves on the skin for liver spots (a fungal skin infection) is a common practice.

Laxative:

The plant is used as a natural laxative.

A clinical trial in Thailand reported the leaf extract as being effective as a laxative.

Other Potential Benefits:

Antibacterial, antimicrobial, antifungal, analgesic, and anti-inflammatory properties.

May help reduce blood pressure, as suggested by studies in Jamaica.

May help reduce sticky blood and plaque buildup in arteries, due to the presence of adenine.

Benefits of Cassia Alata

Natural Skin Remedy: With strong antifungal and antibacterial properties, Cassia alata has long been used to address skin issues such as eczema, ringworm, and fungal infections, promoting a clear and healthy complexion.

Immune Support: Valued for its immune-boosting benefits, this herb helps protect the body from environmental stressors, supporting a resilient immune system.

Liver and Kidney Health: Cassia alata is known for its potential to support liver and kidney function, promoting natural detoxification and assisting these vital organs in the removal of impurities.

Detoxifying Properties: By aiding in the body's natural detox processes, Cassia alata promotes overall well-being and internal balance.

To make King of the Forest tea (also known as Senna alata tea),

- simply steep dried or fresh King of the Forest leaves in boiling water, then simmer, and add honey or sugar to taste.

Shameplant

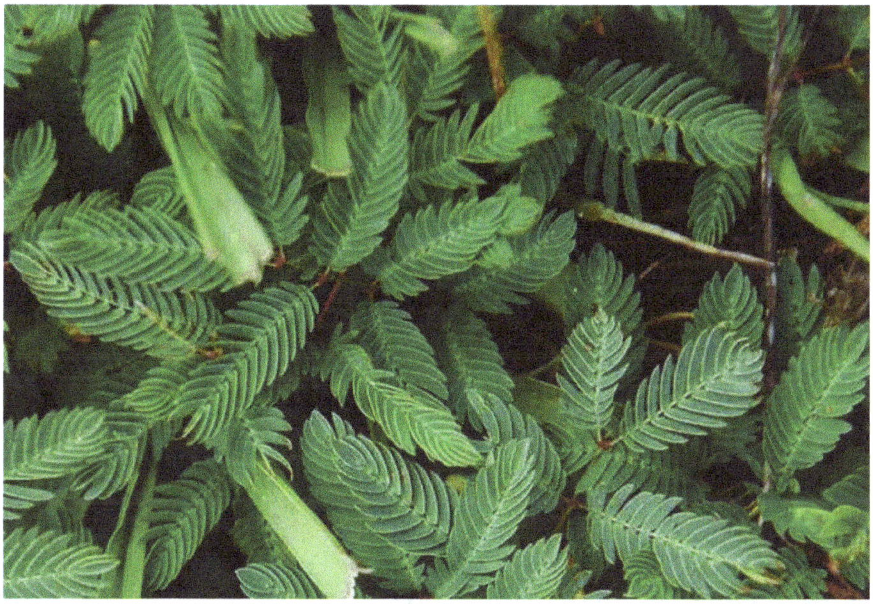

The shameplant (Mimosa pudica), also known as the touch-me-not plant, has several traditional medicinal benefits. It is widely used in herbal medicine for its anti-inflammatory, antimicrobial, and pain-relieving properties. Here are some key benefits:

1. Wound Healing & Skin Care

The leaves and roots have antibacterial properties that help treat wounds, cuts, and skin infections. It can be used to soothe skin irritation and rashes.

2. Pain Relief & Anti-Inflammatory

Acts as a natural painkiller for conditions like arthritis and muscle pain.
Reduces swelling and inflammation in injuries.

3. Digestive Health

Used to treat stomach ulcers and digestive issues.
Helps with diarrhea and intestinal worms.

4. Anxiety & Sleep Aid

Contains sedative properties that help with insomnia and anxiety.
Used in herbal teas to promote relaxation and restful sleep.

5. Blood Sugar Control

Some studies suggest it may help lower blood sugar levels, beneficial for diabetes management.

6. Respiratory Health

Helps relieve asthma and cough due to its expectorant properties.

7. Urinary Tract & Kidney Health

Used in traditional medicine to treat urinary tract infections (UTIs) and kidney-related issues.

How to Make Shameplant (Mimosa pudica) Tea

Ingredients:

- 1–2 teaspoons of dried Mimosa pudica leaves (or fresh leaves)
- 1 cup of water
- Honey or lemon (optional, for taste)

Instructions:

1. Boil the Water – Bring 1 cup of water to a boil.
2. Add the Leaves – Place the dried or fresh leaves in a teacup or teapot.
3. Steep – Pour the hot water over the leaves and let it steep for 5–10 minutes.
4. Strain – Remove the leaves using a strainer.

Serve & Enjoy – Drink warm. You can add honey or lemon if desired.

Health Benefits:

Helps with anxiety and promotes sleep

Supports digestion and relieves stomach discomfort

Aids in reducing inflammation

Hibiscus

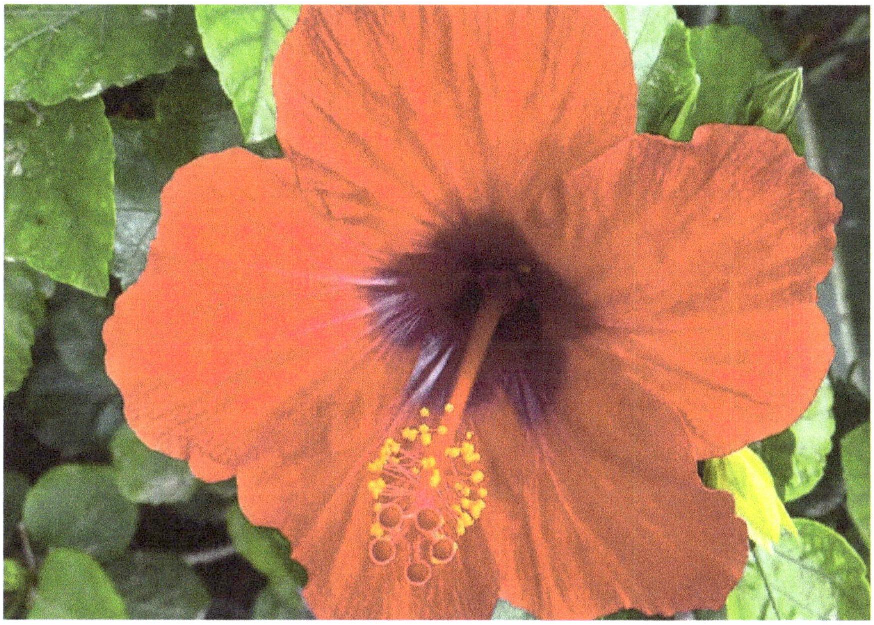

Hibiscus, particularly in tea form, offers numerous health benefits, including supporting heart health by potentially lowering blood pressure, acting as an antioxidant, and potentially aiding in weight loss.

Here's a more detailed look at the potential benefits of hibiscus:

- Heart Health
- Lowering Blood Pressure
- Studies suggest that hibiscus tea can help lower blood pressure, which is beneficial for people with hypertension.
- Supporting Cardiovascular Health
- Hibiscus may contribute to a healthy heart and circulatory system by supporting healthy blood pressure and cholesterol levels.

Antioxidant Properties:

- Rich in Antioxidants
- Hibiscus is packed with antioxidants that help combat oxidative stress and free radicals in the body, potentially reducing the risk of chronic diseases.

Anti-inflammatory Effects:

- The antioxidants in hibiscus may also have anti-inflammatory properties, potentially aiding in reducing swelling and discomfort.

Weight Management:

- Hibiscus tea may help with weight management by boosting metabolism, suppressing appetite, and promoting the elimination of excess water.

Diuretic Properties:

- Hibiscus has diuretic properties, which can help reduce water retention and promote a sense of lightness.

Other Potential Benefits:

Liver Health:

- Hibiscus may help protect the liver from toxins and even demonstrate some anti-cancer activity in laboratory tests of liver cells.

Antibacterial and Antimicrobial Properties:

- Hibiscus tea may have antibacterial and antimicrobial properties that can help to inhibit the growth of bacteria and fight off disease and illness.

Blood Sugar Regulation:

- Hibiscus may help stabilize blood sugar levels, making it a beneficial drink for those looking to control their blood sugar, particularly in the context of a diet aimed at preventing diabetes.

Immunity Boosting:

- Hibiscus may help boost immunity by stimulating B and T cells that have infection-fighting properties.

Hibiscus tea (Ingredients) :

- 1–2 tablespoons of dried hibiscus petals (or 4–5 fresh petals)
- 2 cups of water
- Honey or sugar (optional)
- Lemon or lime (optional, for extra flavor)
- Cinnamon or ginger (optional, for added health benefits)

Vitex/Chaste tree

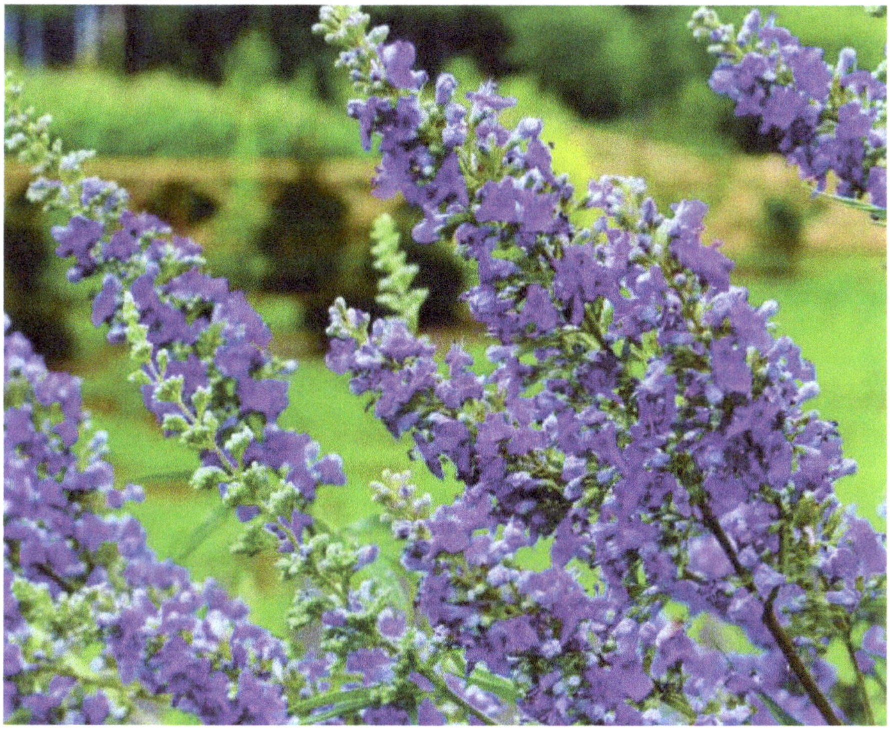

Vitex (Vitex agnus-castus), also known as chaste tree or chasteberry, is a shrub found in the Mediterranean. It is used as a supplement to help alleviate symptoms of premenstrual syndrome, menopause, and polycystic ovary syndrome, and improve fertility.

Health Benefits of Chaste Tree (Vitex agnus-castus)

The Chaste Tree, also known as Vitex or Monk's Pepper, is a powerful herb traditionally used to support hormonal balance and reproductive health. Here are its key benefits:

1. Balances Hormones

Helps regulate estrogen and progesterone levels, making it useful for menstrual cycle irregularities. Supports hormonal balance during menopause, reducing hot flashes and mood swings.

2. Relieves PMS Symptoms

Reduces bloating, irritability, and breast tenderness.

3. Supports Fertility

Promotes ovulation in women struggling with infertility.
Helps treat luteal phase defects, which can impact conception.

4. Reduces Acne

Its hormone-balancing effects may help clear hormonal acne, especially in women.

5. Eases Menopause Symptoms

May reduce hot flashes, night sweats, and mood swings.

6. Supports Prostate Health in Men

Traditionally used to help regulate testosterone levels and reduce an enlarged prostate.

7. Improves Mood & Brain Function

May have a mild dopamine-boosting effect, helping with depression and focus.

How to make Chaste tree tea:

Instructions:

- Crush the berries: Use a mortar and pestle or the back of a spoon to gently crush the dried berries. This helps release their properties.
- Boil the water: Bring 1–2 cups of water to a boil.
- Steep the berries: Place the crushed berries in a teapot or cup and pour the boiling water over them.
- Steep for 10–15 minutes: Cover the cup or teapot to keep in the heat and allow the tea to draw properly.
- Strain: After steeping, strain out the berries.
- Sweeten (optional): Add a little honey or lemon if desired.
- Drink: Best taken once daily, usually in the morning.

Duck Flower

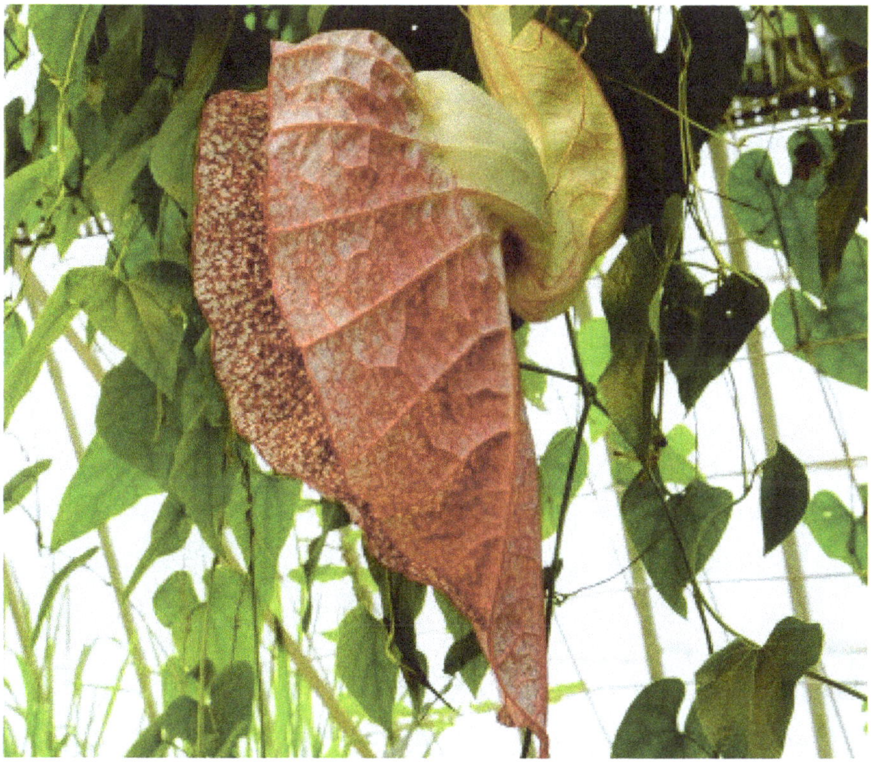

Health Benefits of Aristolochia grandiflora (Duck Flower)
Aristolochia grandiflora, commonly known as the Duck Flower, is a powerful detoxifying herb widely used in traditional medicine, particularly in the Caribbean and Central America. It is known for its intense cleansing effects on the body.

Key Health Benefits:

1. Powerful Detox & Cleanse

- Helps flush out toxins, mucus, and waste from the body.
- Often used for colon and liver cleansing.

2. Boosts Digestive Health

- May help relieve constipation and bloating.
- Supports gut health by removing harmful parasites and bacteria.

3. Increases Energy Levels

- Many users report feeling rejuvenated and energetic after detoxing with duck flower.

4. Supports Weight Loss

- Its detoxifying effects can help remove excess waste and water retention, aiding in weight loss.

5. Strengthens the Immune System

- Helps eliminate toxins and mucus, improving overall immunity.

6. Improves Respiratory Health

- Used to clear excess mucus from the lungs, helping with colds, flu, and congestion.

7. To treat HIV (AIDS)

How to Use Duck Flower for HIV (AIDS)
Dried or Fresh Flower: Consumed as a tea or infusion.

Soaking Method:

Some people soak the flower in water before consumption.
Dried and crushed, soak in warm water for 5-10 minutes. strain and drink, a strong purgative. Repeat every 6 months until symptoms of the virus subside

Caution:

Strong detox effects – can cause nausea, diarrhea, or fatigue during the cleansing process.
Not recommended for pregnant women or people with weak digestion.
Always consult a health professional before use.

Red Raspberry Leaf

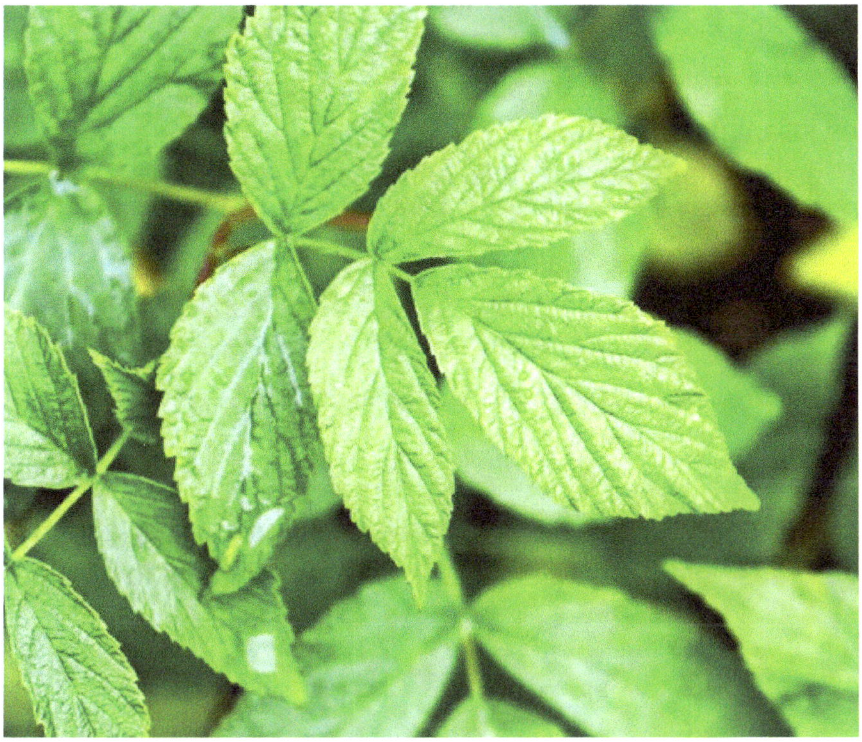

Health Benefits of Red Raspberry Leaf (Rubus idaeus)
Red raspberry leaf is a popular herbal remedy known for its women's health benefits, especially during pregnancy and menstruation. It is rich in vitamins, minerals, and antioxidants that support overall wellness.

1. Supports Women's Reproductive Health

- Helps regulate menstrual cycles and relieve PMS symptoms.
- Reduces cramps, bloating, and heavy periods due to its muscle-relaxing properties.

2. Pregnancy & Labor Support

- Traditionally used to strengthen the uterus and prepare for childbirth.
- May help shorten labor time and reduce complications.
- Supports postpartum recovery and breast milk production.

3. Rich in Nutrients

- Contains iron, calcium, magnesium, potassium, and B vitamins, essential for energy and overall health.
- High in antioxidants, which protect against cell damage.

4. Aids Digestion & Gut Health

- Soothes nausea, bloating, and diarrhea.
- Supports a healthy gut by reducing inflammation.

5. Anti-Inflammatory & Immune Boosting

- Helps reduce inflammation in the body.
- Strengthens the immune system with its antibacterial and antiviral properties.

How to make Red Raspberry Leaf tea

- Tea: Steep 1–2 teaspoons of dried leaves in hot water for 10–15 minutes. Drink 1–3 cups daily.
- Capsules or Tinctures: Available in health stores for convenient use.

Caution:

Pregnant women should consult a doctor before use, especially in early pregnancy. May increase uterine contractions, so best used in the third trimester.

Jewelweed

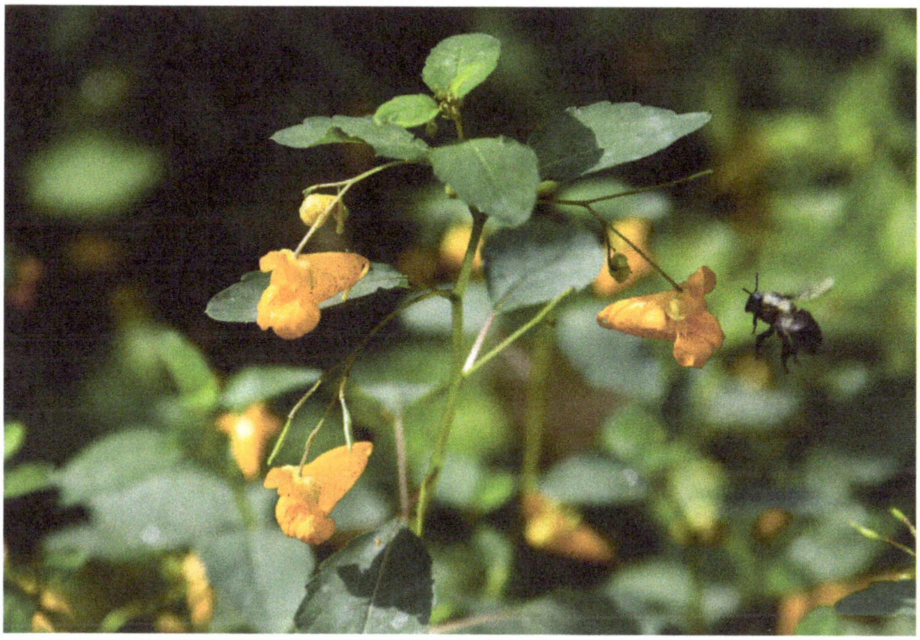

The jewelweed flower's cornucopia-like shape is especially attractive to wildlife like bees, butterflies and hummingbirds, allowing easy access to nectar. (Will Parson/Chesapeake Bay Program)

When spending your day outdoors, you never know what to expect.

Especially in the spring and summer when poisonous plants such as poison ivy are most active (remember, hydrocortisone is an essential addition to your first aid kit!) But what happens if you forget your kit at home? Don't panic! Look around for an orange, spotted, cornucopia-shaped flower—it might just save the day.

Growing anywhere from two to five feet tall, jewelweed is a natural remedy to poison ivy—if you can catch it quickly enough. To use its medicinal properties to prevent a rash, you must apply jewelweed to the infected areas before your immune system can recognize the urushiol oil (what causes the poison ivy rash). This varies by person but can take as little as 10 minutes.

Lucky for you, jewelweed is native to northern and eastern North America and can be found all throughout the Chesapeake Bay watershed. This plant thrives in moist, semi-shady areas, floodplain forests and around forested edges of marshes and bogs—the same areas where poison ivy grows.

Use

Jewelweed is most commonly known for its use in the topical treatment of poison ivy rash due to its antipruritic properties. Various plant parts have traditionally been used orally to promote blood flow, to relieve postchildbirth and joint pain, to treat bruises and swelling, and as an antidote to fish poisoning.

Dosing

Crushed jewelweed has been used as a topical salve for poison ivy; however, no specific dose has been determined in clinical trials.

How to make Jewelweed tea

- Harvest responsibly: Use healthy, non-wilted jewelweed from a clean, pesticide-free area.
- Rinse thoroughly: Clean the plant material under cool running water.
- Chop the stems and leaves roughly to help release their juices.
- Boil: Put the chopped jewelweed in a pot with water and bring to a boil.
- Simmer: Reduce the heat and simmer for about 20–30 minutes. The water should turn a golden orange or amber color.
- Strain: Remove the plant material and let the liquid cool.
- Store: Pour into a glass jar or bottle and refrigerate. It keeps for about 1 week in the fridge, or you can freeze it in ice cube trays for longer storage.

How to use for rashes:

- Dab directly on rashes, bug bites, or areas affected by poison ivy.
- Soak a cloth in the cooled tea and apply it as a compress.
- Add to a spray bottle and mist on the skin.

Feverfew

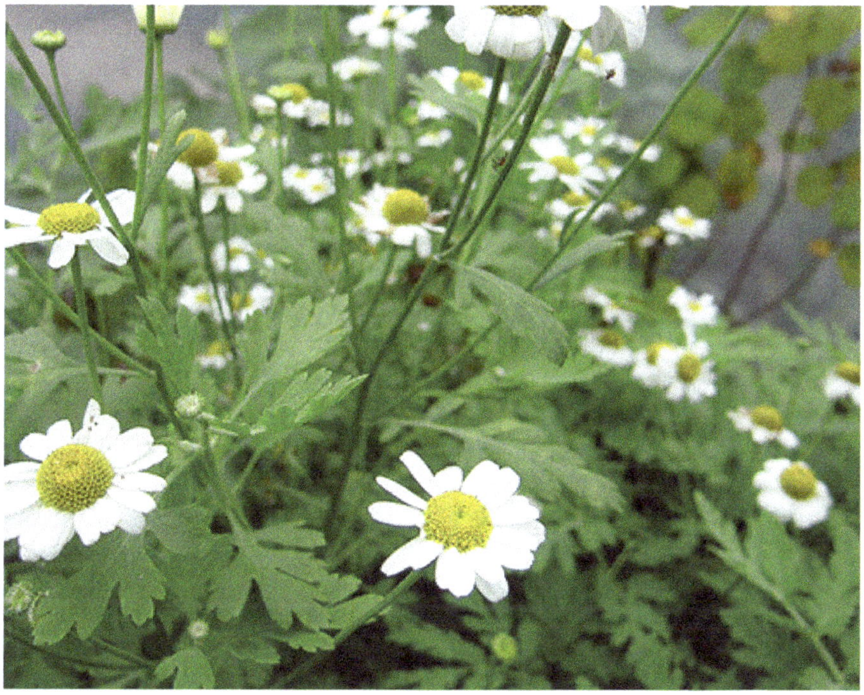

a plant in the daisy family traditionally used for its medicinal properties, particularly for migraine prevention and potentially for other conditions.
Feverfew is a perennial plant with leaves that look like those of chrysanthemum and flowers that look like daisies. Feverfew is native to parts of western Asia and the Balkans, but it now grows throughout the world.

What Is Feverfew?

- A perennial herb native to Europe, now grown worldwide.
- Belongs to the daisy family (Asteraceae).
- Known for its bitter, pungent leaves and medicinal properties.
- Often used dried, fresh, or as capsules, teas, or tinctures.

Migraine Prevention

- Feverfew is best known for reducing the frequency and severity of migraines.
- It doesn't usually stop a migraine in the moment, but works when taken regularly over time.
- The active compound parthenolide is thought to help by calming inflammation and preventing blood vessel spasms.

To use fresh feverfew for migraine prevention or treatment, you can consume it as a tea or chew on the leaves, but it's best to consult with a healthcare professional first, especially if you have any existing medical conditions or take medications.

Preparation and Consumption:

Tea:

- Fresh Leaves: Use 3 teaspoons of fresh feverfew leaves for every cup of boiling water.
- Steep: Let the leaves steep for 5-15 minutes, then strain and serve hot or iced.
- Taste: Feverfew tea can be slightly bitter, so you may want to add honey or other sweeteners to taste.

Chewing the leaves

Fresh Leaves: Some people choose to chew on fresh feverfew leaves, but this can cause mouth irritation.

Start Slowly: If you choose to chew, start with a small amount and gradually increase as needed.

Stinging Nettle

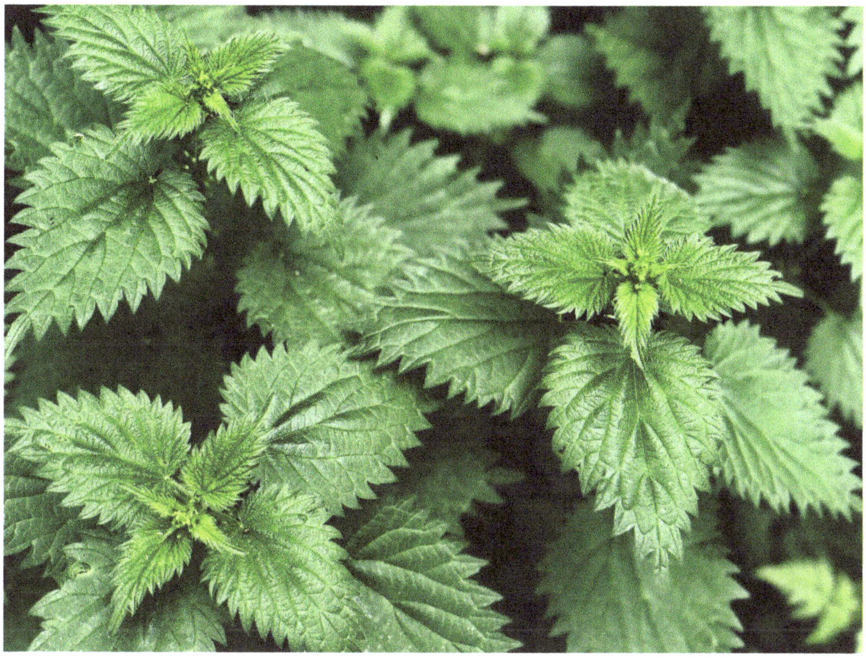

Stinging nettle (Urtica dioica) is a powerful herb with numerous health benefits. Here are some of the most well-known:

1. Anti-Inflammatory Properties

Helps reduce inflammation, making it useful for conditions like arthritis and joint pain. May relieve symptoms of autoimmune diseases like rheumatoid arthritis.

2. Supports Prostate Health

May help with symptoms of benign prostatic hyperplasia (BPH), such as frequent urination. Often used in herbal treatments for prostate enlargement.

3. Allergy Relief (Antihistamine Effects)

Natural antihistamine that may help with hay fever and seasonal allergies. Reduces symptoms like sneezing, itching, and nasal congestion

4. Supports Kidney & Urinary Health

Acts as a diuretic, helping to flush out toxins. May help prevent kidney stones and urinary tract infections (UTIs).

5. Regulates Blood Sugar

May lower blood sugar levels, making it beneficial for diabetes management.

6. Rich in Nutrients

High in vitamins (A, C, K, B-complex), minerals (iron, calcium, magnesium, and potassium), and antioxidants.

Can help with anemia and boost overall energy.

7. Promotes Hair Growth

Improves scalp circulation, potentially reducing hair loss and dandruff.

8. Supports Heart Health

May lower blood pressure and improve circulation.

Contains compounds that help reduce oxidative stress in blood vessels.

9. Aids in Digestion

Helps with bloating, constipation, and gastrointestinal issues.

10. Strengthens the Immune System

Packed with antioxidants that protect against free radicals and infections.

How to Use Stinging Nettle

- **Tea:** Steep dried nettle leaves in hot water.
- **Capsules/Powder**: Found in health stores as supplements.
- **Tinctures**: Liquid extracts for stronger effects.
- **Topical Applications**: Used in creams for joint pain or scalp treatments.

Okra

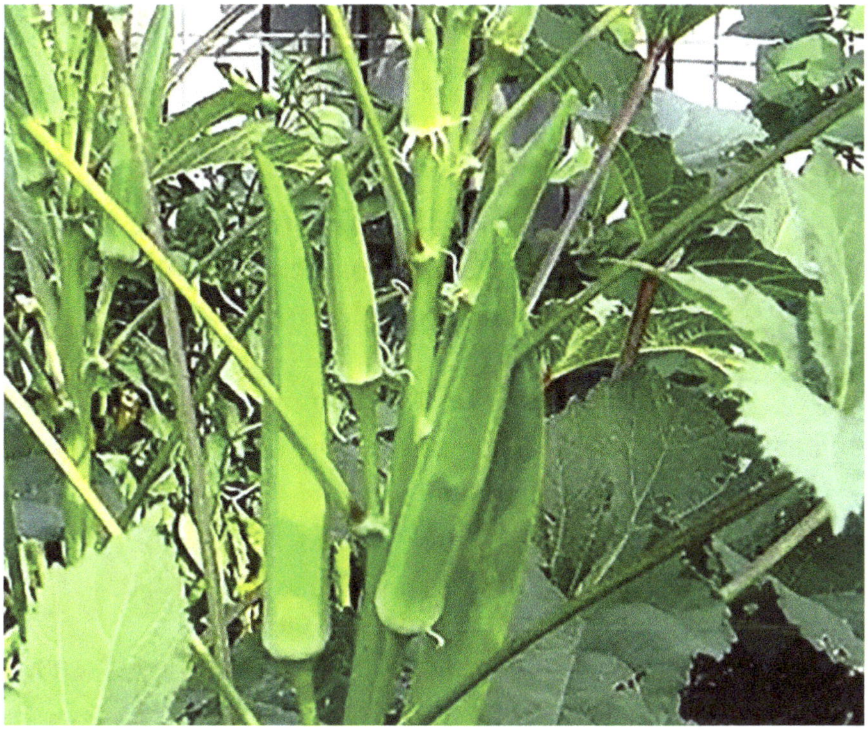

Okra (Abelmoschus esculentus), also known as "lady's finger," is a nutrient-rich vegetable with many health benefits. Here are some of its key advantages:

1. Supports Digestive Health

High in fiber, which promotes healthy digestion and prevents constipation.
Contains mucilage, a gel-like substance that soothes the digestive tract.

2. Helps Control Blood Sugar

May improve insulin sensitivity and regulate blood sugar levels, making it beneficial for diabetes management.
The fiber slows glucose absorption, preventing sugar spikes.

3. Boosts Heart Health

Rich in antioxidants that reduce oxidative stress and lower bad cholesterol (LDL).
Helps maintain healthy blood pressure levels.

4. Supports Weight Management

Low in calories and high in fiber, keeping you full longer and reducing cravings.

5. Strengthens the Immune System

High in vitamin C and antioxidants that boost immunity and fight infections.

6. Promotes Healthy Skin

Vitamin C and antioxidants help reduce skin damage, wrinkles, and inflammation. Keeps skin hydrated and supports collagen production.

7. Improves Eye Health

Rich in vitamin A and beta-carotene, which support good vision and protect against eye diseases.

8. Good for Pregnancy

Contains folate (vitamin B9), which is essential for fetal development and reduces the risk of birth defects.

9. Supports Kidney Health

Helps flush out toxins and reduces the risk of kidney disease.

10. Reduces Inflammation

Contains flavonoids and polyphenols that help reduce inflammation and pain.

How to Use Okra for Health

- Raw or Cooked: Add to soups, stews, stir-fries, or eat it raw in salads.
- Okra Water: Soak chopped okra in water overnight and drink it in the morning for blood sugar and digestion benefits.
- Okra Powder: Used in smoothies or as a supplement.

Contains Lectin (Anti-Cancer Properties)

Studies suggest that lectin, a protein found in okra, may help inhibit the growth of cancer cells. Research on breast cancer cells has shown that okra extract can slow tumor growth.

Okra is rich in folate (Vitamin B9), which helps in DNA synthesis and repair, reducing the risk of DNA mutations that can lead to cancer.

How to Use Okra for Cancer Prevention

- Okra Water: Soak chopped okra in water overnight and drink it in the morning.
- Raw or Cooked: Add to soups, stews, stir-fries, or eat it raw in salads.
- Smoothies: Blend with other anti-cancer foods like turmeric, ginger, and green vegetables.

Bougainvillea

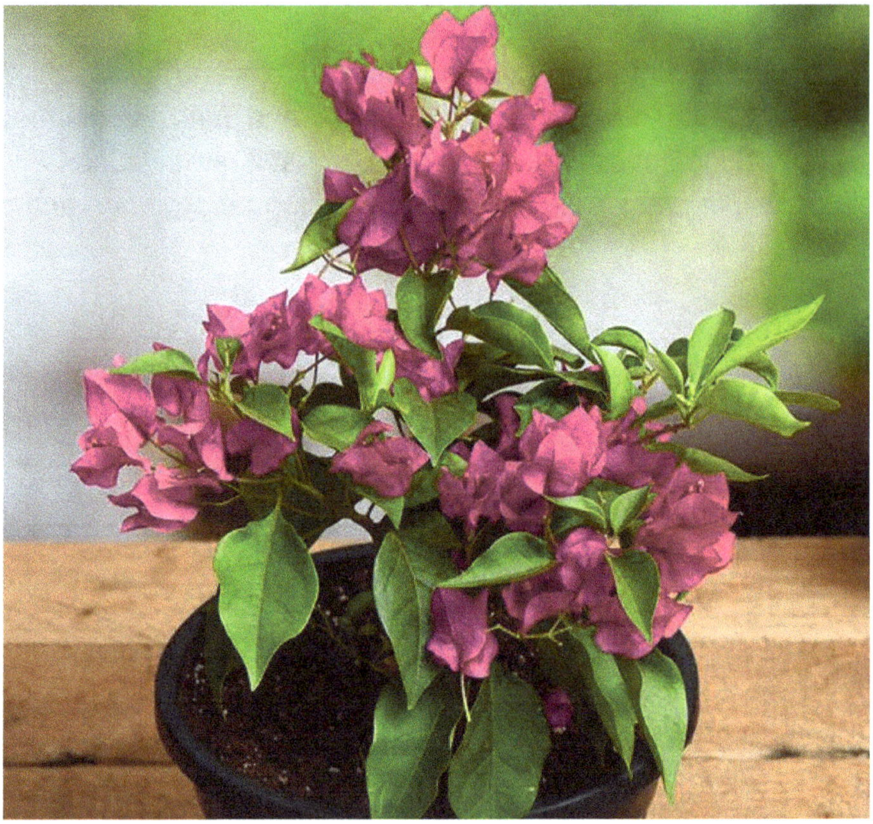

Bougainvillea, particularly Bougainvillea glabra and Bougainvillea spectabilis, has been traditionally used in medicine and is believed to have anti-inflammatory, antioxidant, and antimicrobial properties, potentially aiding in the treatment of respiratory and gastrointestinal issues, as well as supporting blood sugar metabolism.

Here's a more detailed look at the potential health benefits:

Respiratory Issues:
Bougainvillea has been used traditionally to treat coughs, asthma, and bronchitis, likely due to its anti-inflammatory properties.

Gastrointestinal Problems:
Some traditional uses suggest bougainvillea can help with gastrointestinal issues.

Blood Sugar Metabolism:
Bougainvillea spectabilis contains pinitol, which has an insulin-like effect and may help support blood sugar metabolism.

Antioxidant Properties:

Bougainvillea contains phytochemicals like flavonoids and phenolic compounds, which have antioxidant activity, potentially protecting against cell damage.

Antimicrobial Activity:

Bougainvillea has shown antimicrobial and antibiofilm activity, suggesting potential benefits in fighting infections.

Antifungal Activity:

Bougainvillea has been shown to have antifungal activity.

Anti-inflammatory Properties:

Bougainvillea is believed to have anti-inflammatory properties, which could be beneficial for various conditions.

Insecticidal Properties:

Bougainvillea glabra has been found to have important properties as a botanical insecticide.

Bougainvillea tea is a traditional herbal remedy often used for soothing coughs, colds, and respiratory discomfort. It's light, floral, and easy to make. Here's how you can do it:

Ingredients:

- 5–6 fresh or dried bougainvillea petals (make sure they are pesticide-free and well washed)
- 2 cups of water
- 1–2 teaspoons of honey (optional)
- A slice of lemon or a few drops of lemon juice (optional)

Instructions:

1. If using fresh petals, rinse them thoroughly in cold water.
2. If using dried petals, just ensure they are clean and dry.
3. Boil the water:
4. Bring 2 cups of water to a boil in a pot.
5. Add petals:
6. Once the water is boiling, add the bougainvillea petals.
7. Reduce the heat and let them simmer for 5–10 minutes. The water will turn a pinkish or light purple hue.

Mimosa Tree

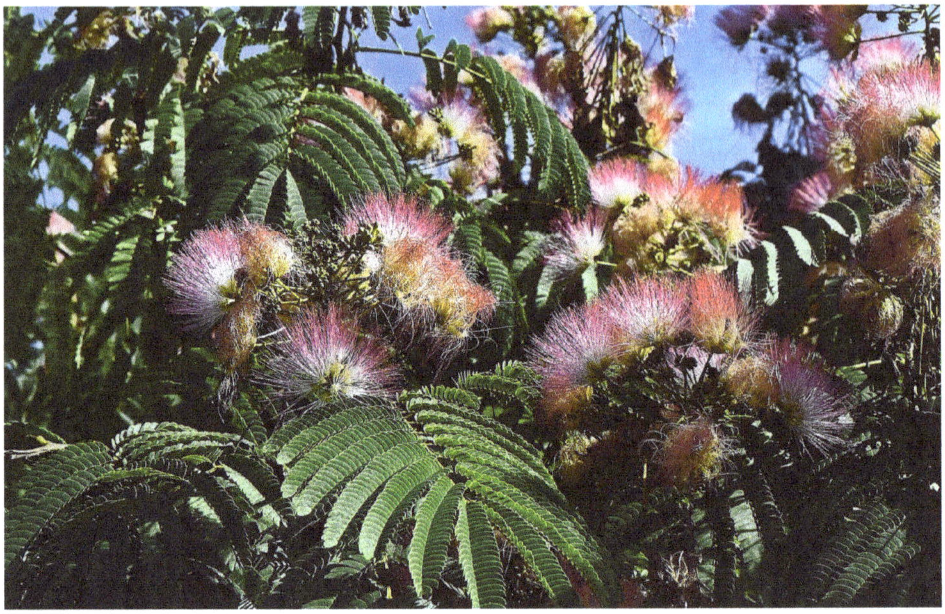

Health Benefits of Mimosa Tree (Albizia julibrissin):
Mood Booster & Natural Antidepressant
Known as the "happiness tree" in Traditional Chinese Medicine.
Used to calm anxiety, reduce stress, and uplift the spirit.

Helps with Insomnia

Mimosa flower and bark are often used in teas or tinctures to promote restful sleep.
Naturally sedative properties without being too strong or addictive.
Supports Emotional Balance
Traditionally used to ease feelings of grief, sadness, and emotional tension.

Anti-inflammatory Properties

Contains antioxidants and anti-inflammatory compounds that may help reduce swelling and inflammation in the body.

Skin Healing & Wound Care

The bark has been used for treating minor wounds, burns, and skin irritations thanks to its antibacterial properties.

Mimosa flower tea is often used as a gentle, natural sedative to help with insomnia and restless sleep.

How it's commonly used:

- Dried bark tea or tincture
- Flower-infused tea
- Powdered bark in capsules
- Topical ointments for wounds

How to Make Mimosa Flower Tea

- 1–2 teaspoons dried mimosa flowers
- 1 cup hot water
- (Optional) Honey or lemon for taste

Instructions:

1. Boil water: Heat 1 cup of water to just below boiling.
2. Steep flowers: Place the dried mimosa flowers in a cup or teapot and pour the hot water over them.
3. Steep for 5–10 minutes: Cover and let the tea steep to draw out the calming properties.
4. Strain & serve: Strain the flowers and enjoy. Add honey or lemon if desired.

Caution:

Should not be taken during pregnancy.
Always use in moderation and consult a healthcare provider before use if you're on medication or have health conditions.

Damiana

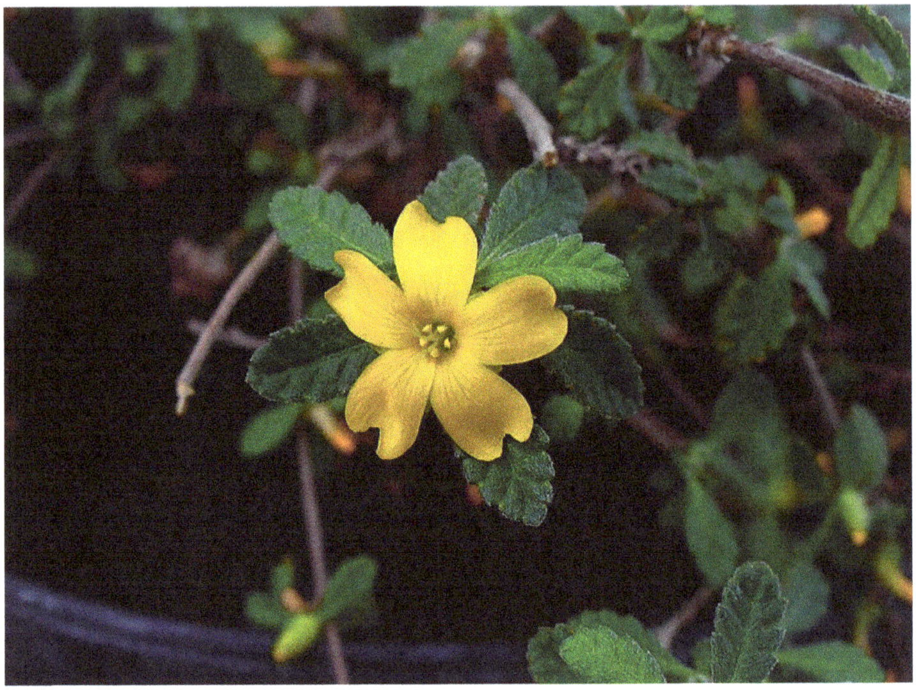

Damiana Health Benefits (Turnera diffusa)

Damiana is a small shrub native to Mexico, Central America, and the Caribbean, traditionally used as an herbal remedy for centuries. It's known for its slightly sweet, aromatic leaves and has gained popularity for both physical and emotional wellness.

Natural Aphrodisiac

Damiana is most famous for enhancing libido in both men and women.
It may help with sexual stamina and sensitivity, and has been traditionally used to boost desire and intimacy.

Mood and Stress Relief

Known to have mild antidepressant and anti-anxiety properties.
Helps calm the nerves, reduce stress, and promote emotional balance.

Energy and Stamina

Used to combat fatigue and improve overall energy levels without the jitters.

Digestive Support

Traditionally used to relieve constipation, indigestion, and mild gastrointestinal discomfort.

Hormonal Balance

Damiana may help regulate hormonal fluctuations, making it popular among women for menstrual irregularities and menopause symptoms.

Respiratory Health

It can be used as a natural expectorant to help clear the lungs and ease coughing.

Urinary Tract Support

May help soothe mild bladder irritation and support urinary health.

Ways to Use Damiana:

- Tea (steep dried leaves for a calming, mood-lifting drink)
- Tincture or liquid extract
- Capsules or powder
- Smoking blend (sometimes used as a mild herbal relaxant)
- In herbal liqueurs (it's one of the ingredients in traditional Mexican liqueurs)

Making Damiana tea is super easy—and it's one of those herbs with a mystical, sensual, and slightly rebellious vibe. Known for its mood-boosting and aphrodisiac properties, Damiana has been used for centuries in Central and South America for everything from relaxation to romance.

How to Make Damiana Tea

Ingredients

- 1 to 2 teaspoons of dried Damiana leaves
- 1 cup of hot water (not boiling)
- Optional: honey, lemon, or cinnamon for taste

Precautions:

Avoid excessive use; large doses may cause mild hallucinations or nausea.

Not recommended for pregnant or breastfeeding women.

Always consult with a healthcare provider if taking medication or if you have existing health conditions.

Coleus Plant

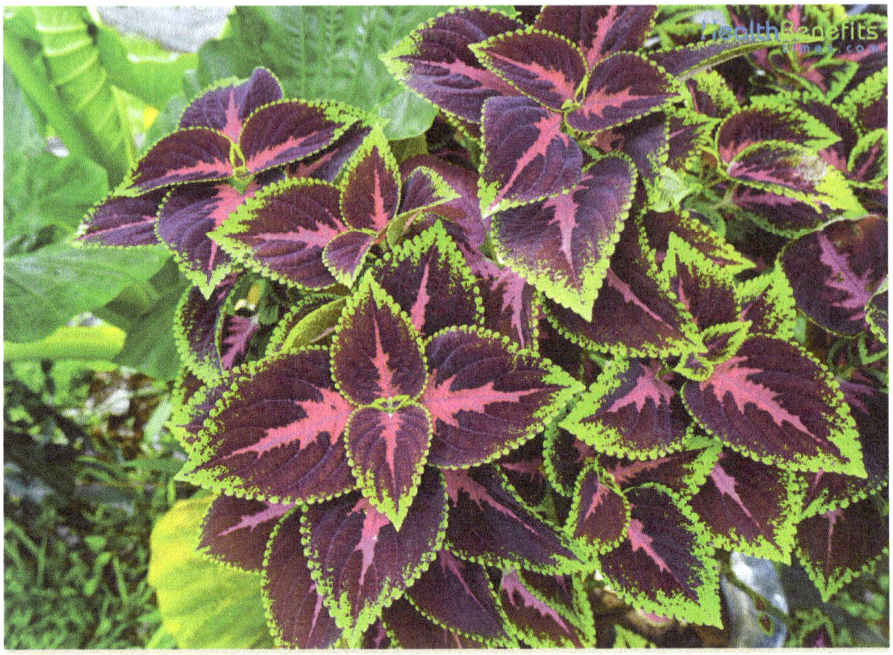

The Coleus plant is a beautiful and vibrant plant known mostly for its stunning foliage rather than flowers. It's a favorite for both gardeners and houseplant lovers due to its easy care and variety of colors and patterns.

Health benefits

Weight Loss Support

- Forskolin is often used in supplements for fat burning and weight management.
- It helps stimulate the production of cyclic AMP (cAMP), which can promote fat breakdown and metabolism.

Heart Health

- Coleus has been used to help lower blood pressure and improve heart function.
- It may help dilate blood vessels and improve blood flow.

Asthma Relief

- Forskolin is a natural bronchodilator, which can help relax airways and reduce asthma symptoms.

Improved Circulation

- The plant has vasodilating effects, which help improve blood circulation and may prevent clot formation.

Glaucoma Management

- Some studies show that forskolin eye drops may help reduce intraocular pressure in people with glaucoma.

To make Coleus tea, simply steep dried Coleus leaves in hot water for 5 minutes, strain, and drink.

Here's a more detailed breakdown:

Gather your ingredients: You'll need dried Coleus leaves and hot water.

- Infuse the leaves: Place 1/2 to 1 teaspoon of dried Coleus leaves into a cup or teapot.
- Pour boiling water: Pour 1 cup of boiling water over the leaves.
- Steep: Allow the leaves to steep for 5 minutes.
- Strain and serve: Strain the tea and enjoy.
- Optional additions: You can add rock sugar or other sweeteners to taste.

Indian Almond Leaf

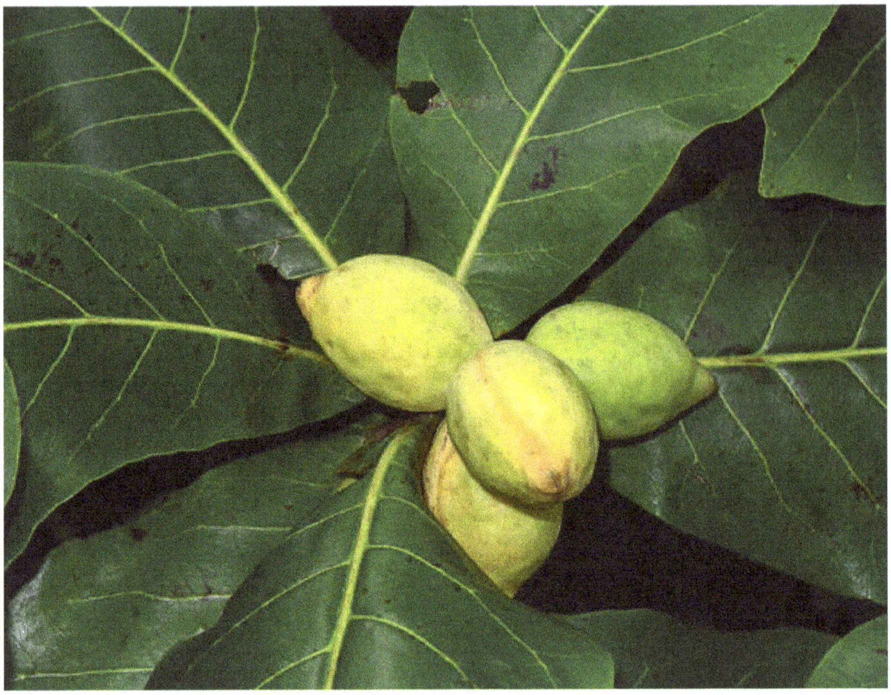

Indian almond leaves are large, tropical leaves from the Terminalia catappa tree, commonly found in Asia, Africa, and the Caribbean. They are famously used in aquariums for fish health — but they also offer several traditional medicinal benefits for humans in herbal remedies.

Top Health Benefits of Indian Almond Leaves:

Anti-inflammatory Properties

- Traditionally used to reduce swelling and soothe inflamed skin.
- Helps relieve skin conditions like rashes, eczema, and minor cuts.

Antioxidant Rich

- Contains flavonoids and tannins that help fight free radicals, supporting overall cellular health and slowing aging.

Anti-bacterial and Anti-fungal

- The leaf extracts are known to inhibit bacteria and fungi, making them useful in herbal skin rinses or topical treatments for infections and wounds.

Liver Protection

- Some traditional practices use Indian almond leaf tea to detoxify and support liver health.

Blood Sugar Regulation

Early research shows potential for helping to manage blood sugar levels, though more studies are needed.

Digestive Support

Traditional use includes relieving diarrhea and digestive discomfort.

Oral Health

In some cultures, the leaves are chewed or used in mouth rinses to help fight gum infections and promote fresh breath.

How It's Commonly Used:

- Herbal tea (dried leaves steeped in hot water)
- Topical washes (for skin irritations and wounds)
- Soaks and baths (for skin inflammation and muscle relaxation)

How to Make Indian Almond Leaf Tea (for human use):

Ingredients:

- 1–2 dried Indian almond leaves
- 2 cups water
- Wash the leaves.
- Boil water and add the leaves.
- Let simmer for 5–7 minutes until the water turns light brown.
- Strain and drink warm. You can add honey if desired.

Precautions:

Avoid excessive use; stick to small doses as part of a balanced herbal routine. Always consult with a healthcare provider before using it medicinally, especially if pregnant or on medication.

Banana Leaf

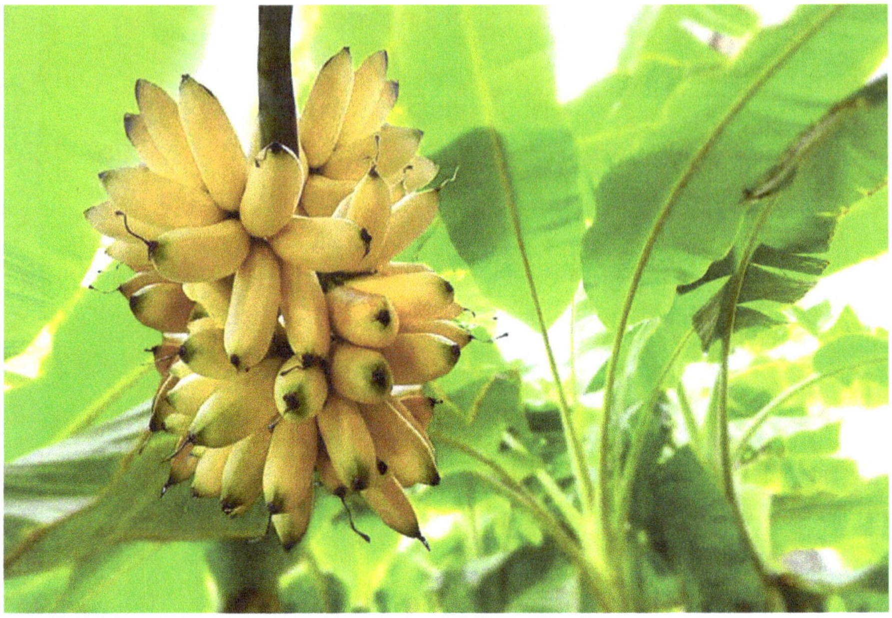

Banana Leaf Tea Health Benefits

Banana leaf tea is made from the leaves of the banana plant, and it's been used in traditional herbal medicine for centuries. The leaves are packed with antioxidants, polyphenols, and other plant compounds that can offer several health benefits.

Top Health Benefits of Banana Leaf Tea

Rich in Antioxidants

- Helps fight free radicals and reduce oxidative stress, which supports overall cellular health and slows aging.

Supports Digestion

- Traditionally used to soothe the stomach, reduce bloating, and aid in smoother digestion.

Boosts Immunity

- The tea is believed to strengthen the immune system thanks to its antioxidant and antibacterial properties.

Anti-inflammatory Effects

- Can help reduce inflammation in the body and may relieve minor aches and pains.

May Help Control Blood Sugar Levels

- Some studies suggest banana leaf compounds could help regulate blood sugar levels and improve insulin sensitivity.

Detoxifying Properties

- The tea is thought to help flush toxins from the body and support liver health.

Skin Health

- Banana leaf has antimicrobial properties that can help promote clearer skin and soothe skin irritation if used externally.

How to Make Banana Leaf Tea:

Ingredients:

- 1–2 fresh or dried banana leaves (washed and cut into small pieces)
- 2 cups water
- Honey or lemon (optional)
- Boil the water.

- Add the banana leaves and let them simmer for 5–7 minutes.
- Strain into a cup.
- Add honey or lemon if desired and enjoy warm!

Precaution:

Always make sure the leaves are well-cleaned and chemical-free.
Start with small amounts if you're trying it for the first time, especially if you have any allergies or health conditions.

Purslane

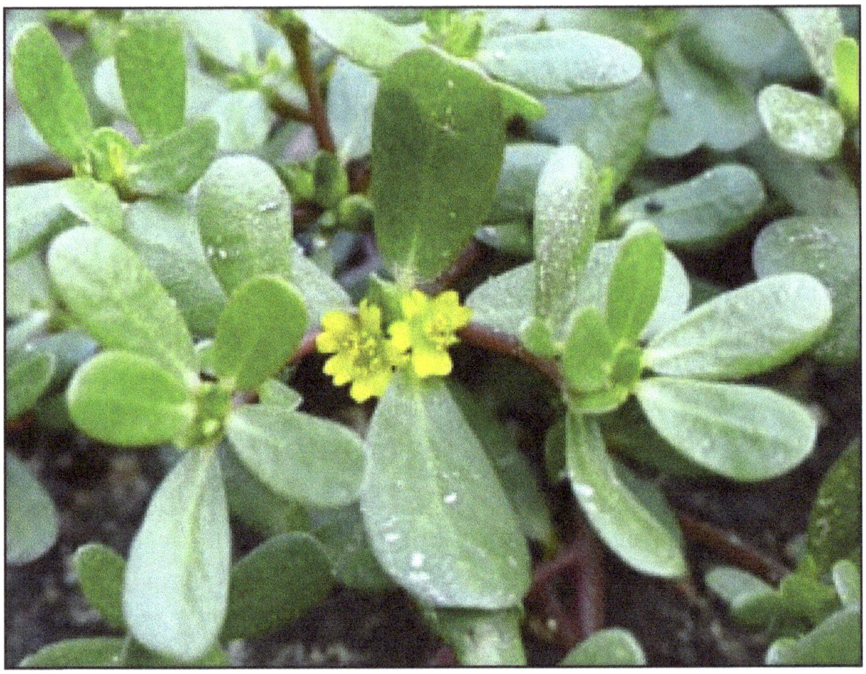

Purslane is a nutritional powerhouse with benefits ranging from improved heart health and diabetes management to antioxidant and anti-inflammatory properties. It's rich in omega-3 fatty acids, vitamins (A, C), and minerals (potassium, magnesium, calcium), making it a valuable addition to a healthy diet.

Specific Benefits

Heart Health:

- Purslane is a good source of omega-3 fatty acids, which can help reduce the risk of heart disease and stroke.

Diabetes Management:

- Some studies suggest purslane may help regulate blood sugar levels and improve lipid profiles, potentially aiding in diabetes management.

Antioxidant and Anti-inflammatory Properties:

Purslane contains antioxidants like beta-carotene and vitamin C, which can help protect against cell damage and reduce inflammation.

Purslane (Portulaca oleracea) is a super underrated wild edible that grows like a weed in many places — but it's actually a nutritional powerhouse! People around the world eat it raw in salads, cooked in soups, or even stir-fried.

Packed with Vitamins & Minerals

- Vitamin A – Good for eyes and immune system.
- Vitamin C – Antioxidant, boosts immunity and skin repair.
- Vitamin E – Skin health and cell protection.
- Magnesium, Potassium, Calcium, and Iron – Great for muscles, bones, and circulation.

High in Antioxidants

- Contains beta-carotene, glutathione, melatonin, and betalain pigments, all of which help fight oxidative stress and protect your cells.
- Supports Blood Sugar Balance
- Some studies suggest purslane may help lower blood sugar levels — helpful for type 2 diabetes management.

Hydrating & Cooling

- Purslane is made up of about 93% water — great for hydration, especially in hot climates.

You can enjoy purslane (Portulaca oleracea) in a bunch of tasty and healthy ways! It's super versatile — you can eat it raw, cooked, or even use it in teas or smoothies. Here's how to consume it:

Raw (Fresh in Salads & Wraps)

Just rinse well and toss into salads — it has a mild, lemony, slightly salty flavor.
Mix with cucumber, tomato, onions, lime juice, and olive oil for a refreshing summer salad.
Add to wraps, sandwiches, or tacos for a crisp, hydrating crunch.

Cooked (Steamed, Stir-Fried, or Soups)

Sauté in olive oil with garlic and onions like spinach.
Add to soups, stews, or curries — especially good in brothy dishes.
Lightly steam it and drizzle with lemon juice and sea salt.

Dandelion

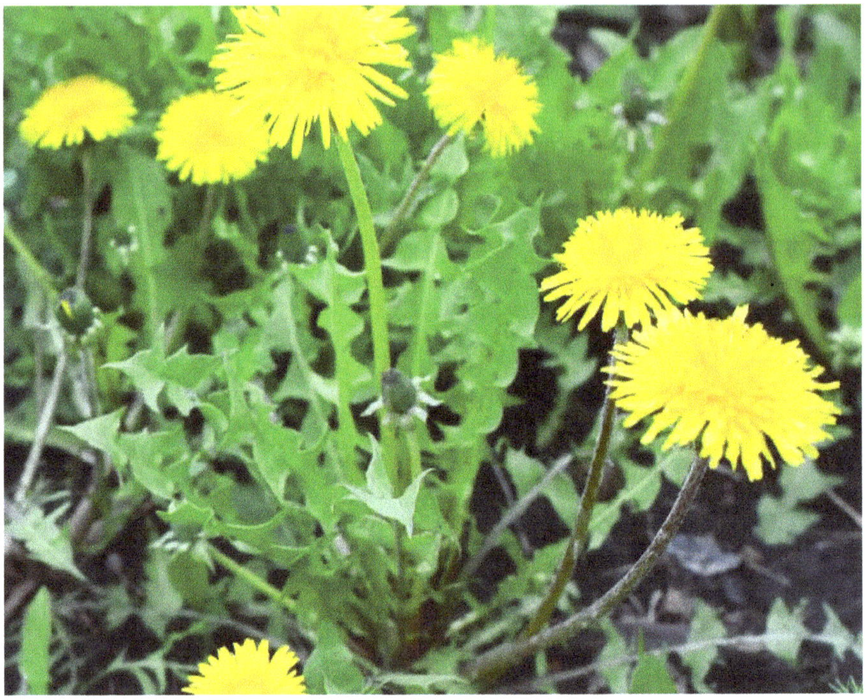

Dandelion leaves, roots, and flowers may offer health benefits. These can include promoting liver health and fighting inflammation.

Although often dismissed as a stubborn lawn weed, people have used dandelion in forms of traditional medicine for centuries.

Not only can the leaves, roots, and flowers add color to your plate, but they're also often found in herbal teas and supplements, where they're used as a natural remedy to support blood sugar management and boost skin, liver, and heart health.

1. Highly nutritious

From root to flower, dandelions are highly nutritious plants loaded with vitamins, minerals, and fiber.

Dandelion greens can be eaten cooked or raw and are an excellent source of vitamins A, C, and K. They also contain vitamin E, folate, and small amounts of other B vitamins. Dandelion greens provide several minerals, including iron, calcium, magnesium, and potassium.

Dandelion root is rich in the carbohydrate inulin, a type of soluble fiber found in plants that supports the growth and maintenance of healthy gut bacteria in your digestive tract. Dandelion root is often dried and made into tea, but you can also eat it whole like other root vegetables.

2. Contains potent antioxidants

Dandelion contains potent antioxidants, which may explain many of its medicinal properties.

Antioxidants are compounds that help neutralize free radicals — molecules that are a product of normal metabolism but contribute to chronic disease risk if levels get too high in your body. Therefore, antioxidants are crucial for your overall health.

Dandelions contain high levels of the antioxidant beta-carotene, which may protect against cell damage and oxidative stress

3. May help fight inflammation

Dandelion may reduce inflammation thanks to compounds such as polyphenols. Inflammation is a natural immune system response to injury or infection. However, long-term inflammation may permanently damage body tissues and DNA.

Some test-tube studies note significantly reduced markers of inflammation in cells treated with compounds extracted from dandelion

4. May aid in blood sugar management

Chicoric and chlorogenic acid are two bioactive compounds in dandelion that may help decrease blood sugar levels. Test-tube and animal studies show that these compounds may improve the secretion of insulin — a hormone that regulates blood sugar levels — and the absorption of glucose (sugar) in your muscles.

This process improves insulin sensitivity and reduces blood sugar levels. Chicoric and chlorogenic acid may also limit the digestion of starchy, high carb foods, which may further contribute to dandelion's ability to lower blood sugar levels.

1. Dandelion Leaf Tea (Best for detox and digestion)

Ingredients:

- 1–2 teaspoons of dried dandelion leaves (or a small handful of fresh leaves)
- 1 cup of hot water
- Honey or lemon (optional)

Instructions:

1. Wash and chop fresh dandelion leaves (if using fresh).
2. Boil 1 cup of water.
3. Pour hot water over the leaves in a cup.
4. Cover and steep for 5–7 minutes.
5. Strain, add honey or lemon if desired, and enjoy.

2. Dandelion Root Tea (Best for liver support and energy boost)

Ingredients:

- 1–2 teaspoons of dried dandelion root (store-bought or harvested, cleaned, dried, and chopped)
- 1 cup water

Instructions:

1. Add dandelion root to water in a small pot.
2. Bring to a gentle boil, then reduce heat and simmer for 10–15 minutes.
3. Strain and pour into a cup.
4. Add honey, cinnamon, or ginger if you like for flavor.

Cassia occidentalis

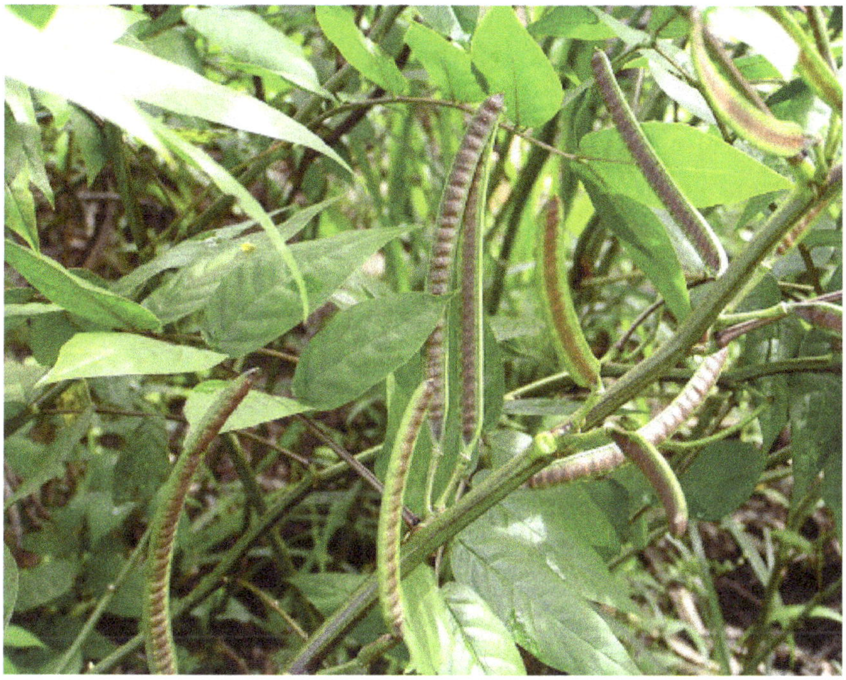

Cassia occidentalis (also known as coffee senna, negro coffee, or septic weed) has been used in traditional herbal medicine in various cultures. Here are some of its health benefits and ways to consume it:

Health Benefits of Cassia occidentalis

Detoxification

- Traditionally used as a mild laxative and body cleanser, helping to detoxify the liver and digestive system.

Improves Digestion

- Helps relieve constipation and promote bowel regularity.
- Anti-inflammatory Properties — Used to reduce inflammation and swelling.

Fever Reduction

- Often used in traditional medicine to help lower fevers.

Immune Support

- Believed to strengthen the immune system.

Relieves Muscle Pain

- Some cultures use it for muscle aches and joint pain relief.

Skin Health

- Used externally as a wash for skin irritations and infections.

Herbal Tea

- Use dried leaves, seeds, or roots.
- Boil 1 teaspoon in 2 cups of water for 5–10 minutes.
- Strain and drink warm.

Powder Form

- The dried seeds or roots can be ground into powder.
- Take 1/4 teaspoon in warm water or mix into smoothies.

Coffee Substitute

- Roasted seeds are often brewed as a coffee alternative (hence the name "negro coffee").
- Roast the seeds, grind, and brew like coffee.

Decoction (for external use)

- Boil leaves or roots in water, cool, and use as a skin wash for rashes or infections.

Caution

Do not overconsume — high doses can cause toxicity.
Avoid during pregnancy without medical advice.
Prolonged use is not recommended without professional supervision.

Piper Umbellatum

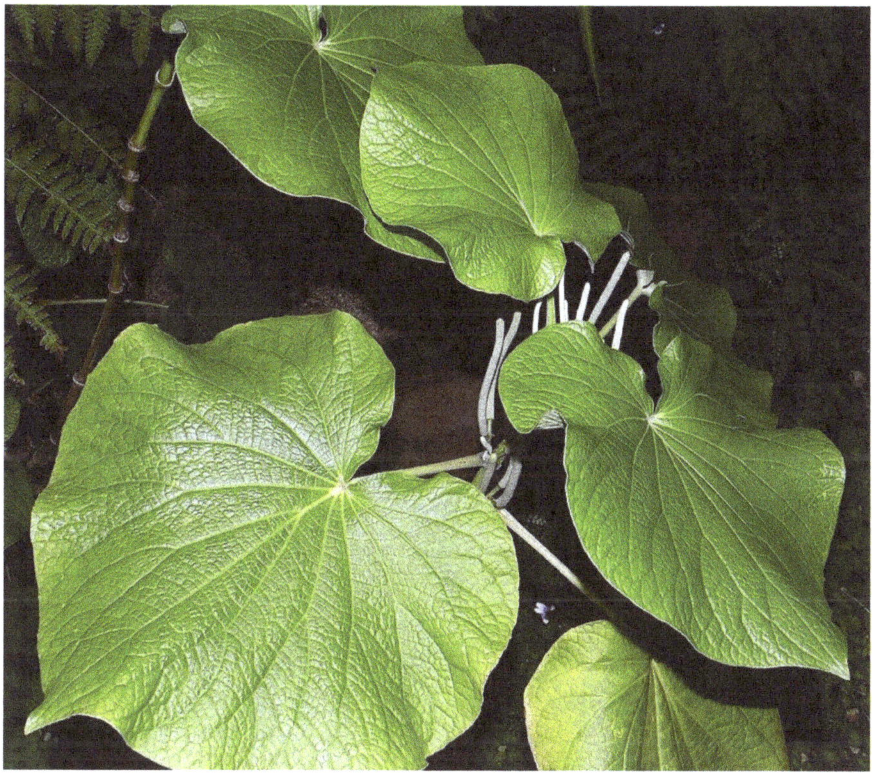

Piper umbellatum, also known as cow's foot leaf, exhibits a wide range of potential benefits, including antibacterial, anti-inflammatory, antioxidant, and gastroprotective properties, with traditional uses for various ailments.

Traditional Uses and Potential Benefits

Folk Medicine

- In traditional herbal medicine, Piper umbellatum is used to treat a variety of conditions, including rheumatism, inflammatory tumors, stomach pains, and ascites.

Antibacterial and Antifungal

- Extracts and compounds from Piper umbellatum have shown antibacterial and antifungal activities.

Antioxidant

- The plant contains compounds with antioxidant properties, which can help protect against cell damage caused by free radicals.
- Anti-inflammatory

Anti-inflammatory

- Piper umbellatum has demonstrated anti-inflammatory effects, potentially useful in treating conditions like inflammatory bowel disease.

Gastroprotective

- Studies suggest that Piper umbellatum can protect against ulcers and promote healing of the stomach lining.

Antimalarial

- Some studies suggest potential antimalarial activity.

Antileishmanial and Antitrypanosomal:

- Research indicates potential activity against leishmaniasis and trypanosomiasis.

Analgesic

- The plant may have pain-relieving properties.

Antidiabetic

- Some studies suggest that extracts from Piper umbellatum can inhibit enzymes involved in diabetes.

Here's a more detailed breakdown of how Piper umbellatum is consumed

Leaves and Inflorescences:

Young leaves and inflorescences are commonly eaten raw in salads or steamed and served as a vegetable.

They can also be used as a condiment with fish, meat, or rice.
In some regions, the leaves are used to wrap other foods during cooking, like in the Filipino dish "pinais" where they wrap steamed shrimp and grated coconut.

Passion flower

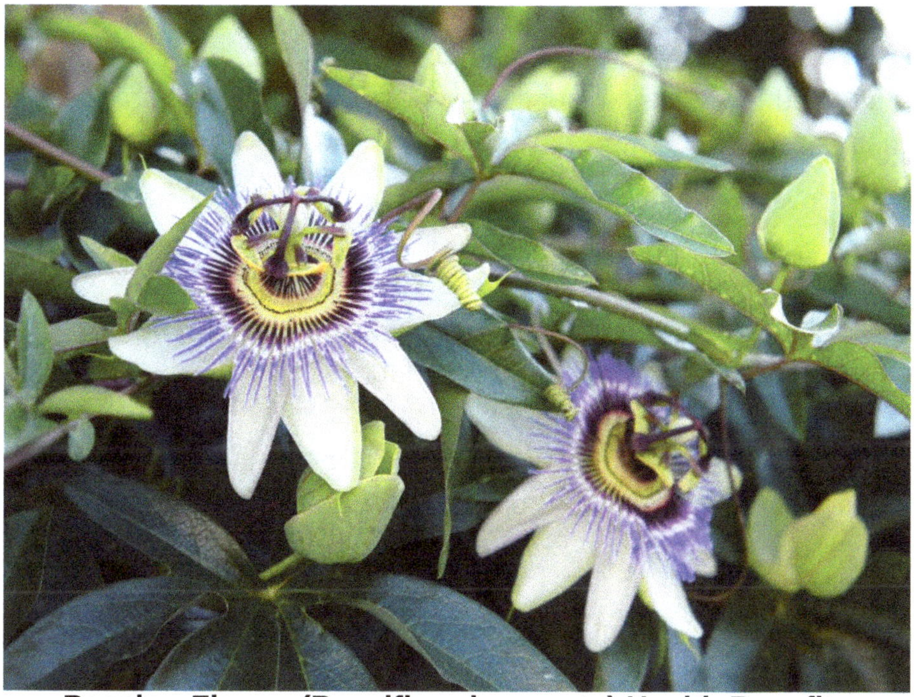

Passion Flower (Passiflora incarnata) Health Benefits

Passion flower is a beautiful climbing vine with calming properties, widely used in herbal medicine for its ability to soothe the mind and body.

Key Health Benefits of Passion Flower

- Relieves Anxiety and Stress
- Passion flower is well-known for its calming effects on the nervous system, helping to reduce anxiety and promote relaxation.

Improves Sleep

- Commonly used as a natural remedy for insomnia and sleep disturbances. It helps induce deeper, restful sleep without leaving grogginess.

Mild Pain Relief

- Some studies show it has mild analgesic (pain-relieving) properties and can help reduce muscle tension or headaches caused by stress.

Menopausal Symptom Relief

- Passion flower may help ease hot flashes, mood swings, and irritability during menopause.

Supports Heart Health

- By helping to lower blood pressure and reduce stress, passion flower may indirectly support cardiovascular health.

Relieves Stomach Discomfort

- It can also be used to calm the digestive system, particularly when stress is the cause of upset stomach.

How to Consume Passion Flower

Herbal Tea

- Steep 1 teaspoon of dried passion flower in hot water for 5–10 minutes.
- Drink 1–2 cups per day, especially before bed for relaxation.

Tincture (liquid extract)

- Use as directed (commonly 10–30 drops in water or juice, 2–3 times daily).

Capsules

- Available in supplement form. Follow dosage instructions on the product label.

Passion Flower Powder

Can be added to smoothies or warm beverages in small amounts.

Precautions

Should not be used in excess — large amounts can cause drowsiness or dizziness.
Not recommended for use with sedative medications or alcohol.
Consult a healthcare provider before use if pregnant, breastfeeding, or on medication.

Shatavari

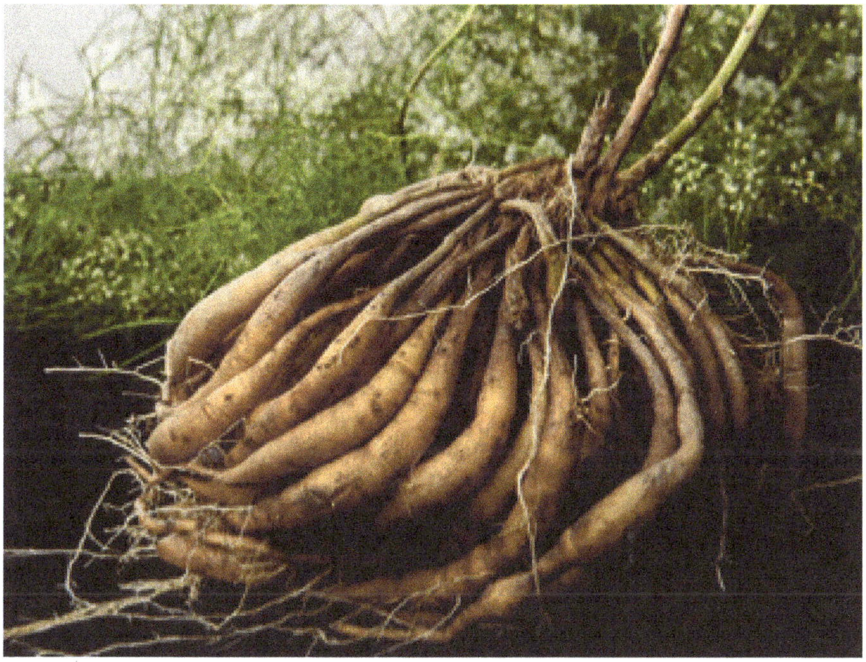

Shatavari is an Ayurvedic rasayana herb which is also known as the female-friendly herb. It is helpful in menstrual disorders and acts as a uterine tonic. It enhances breast development and increases breast milk production by regulating hormonal balance.

Shatavari is also beneficial for men as it improves testosterone levels. It might be good for diabetics as it helps manage blood sugar levels. Shatavari might also promote memory functions due to its antioxidant activity.

According to Ayurveda, Shatavari boosts immunity due to its Rasayana (rejuvenating) property and helps in weight gain due to its Balya property.
Shatavari powder can be taken along with milk or honey twice a day to get relief from the symptoms of premenstrual syndrome.

Applying Shatavari powder paste along with milk or honey on the skin helps to get rid of wrinkles. It can also help promote wound healing when applied along with coconut oil. People with weak digestion are advised to avoid taking Shatavari as it is Guru (heavy) in nature and might take time to get digested.

How to Consume Shatavari (Asparagus racemosus)

Shatavari is a revered adaptogenic herb in Ayurvedic medicine, known as the "Queen of Herbs" for its benefits in supporting female reproductive health, hormone balance, digestive health, and immunity. It is also beneficial for men, offering strength, vitality, and stress relief.

How to Consume Shatavari

Shatavari Powder (Churna)

- Dosage: ½ to 1 teaspoon (about 3-6 grams) daily.
- How to take:
- Mix in warm milk, warm water, or herbal tea with honey.
- Traditionally taken with warm milk and a pinch of cardamom at night for hormonal balance and relaxation

Shatavari Capsules/Tablets

- Dosage: As directed on the label (commonly 500–1000 mg, once or twice daily).
- Easy and convenient for daily use, especially for those who dislike the taste of the powder.

- Shatavari Liquid Extract (Tincture)
- Dosage: 20–30 drops in water, 1–2 times a day.
- Quick absorption, good for stress relief and energy.
- Shatavari Ghee (Ayurvedic preparation)

Shatavari is sometimes infused in ghee for deep nourishment.

- 1 teaspoon daily on an empty stomach, or stirred into warm milk or porridge.

Best Times to Take

Morning (on an empty stomach) for energy and vitality.

Night (with warm milk) for hormone balance, stress relief, and better sleep.

Cloves (Kidney Cleanse)

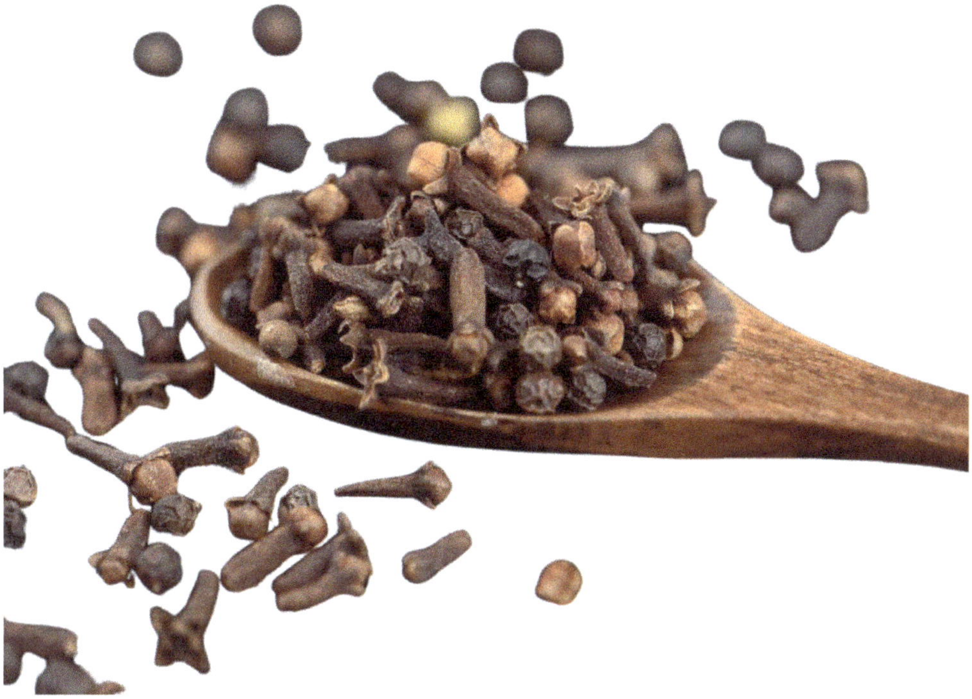

Cloves are a versatile spice that adds flavor while also providing health benefits. They are high in antioxidants, may help regulate blood sugar, kill bacteria, and more.

Cloves are the flower buds of the clove tree, an evergreen also known as Syzygium aromaticum.

Found in both whole and ground forms, this versatile spice can be used to season pot roasts, add flavor to hot beverages, and bring spicy warmth to cookies and cakes.

You may know cloves as one of the main ingredients in gingerbread baked goods or a staple spice in Indian cuisine.
Cloves are best known as a sweet and aromatic spice, but they have also been used in traditional medicine.

In fact, research suggests that the compounds in cloves may have several health benefits, including supporting liver health and helping stabilize blood sugar levels.

Clove is a powerful spice with antioxidant, anti-inflammatory, and antibacterial properties that can support kidney health. While it's not a direct "kidney cleanser," it can help reduce oxidative stress, fight infections, and support overall kidney function. Here's how you can use clove for kidney health:

1. Clove Tea for Kidney Health

Drinking clove tea can help flush out toxins and support kidney function.

Ingredients:

- 3-4 cloves
- 1 cup of hot water
- Honey or lemon (optional)

Instructions:

1. Crush the cloves slightly to release their oils.
2. Add them to a cup of hot water and let steep for 10–15 minutes.
3. Strain and drink once a day, preferably in the morning.

2. Clove Water Detox

- Soaking cloves in water overnight allows their beneficial compounds to infuse into the water.

Instructions:

- Soak 4–5 cloves in a glass of water overnight.
- Drink the infused water on an empty stomach in the morning.
- 3. Clove and Ginger Kidney Cleanse
- Combining clove with ginger enhances its detoxifying effects.

Ingredients:

- 3 cloves
- 1-inch piece of fresh ginger
- 1 cup of hot water

Instructions:

1. Grate the ginger and add it to a cup of hot water along with the cloves.
2. Let it steep for 10–15 minutes.
3. Strain and drink once or twice a day.
4. 4. Clove Oil for Kidney Support
5. Clove oil has antimicrobial properties that can help prevent kidney infections.

How to Use:

Add 1–2 drops of food-grade clove oil to warm water or tea.
Do not consume in excess, as clove oil is very potent.

Precautions:

Avoid excessive consumption, as cloves contain eugenol, which can be harmful in large doses.

If you have kidney disease or take medication, consult your doctor before using clove regularly.
Pregnant and breastfeeding women should use clove in moderation.

Green tea for Lupus

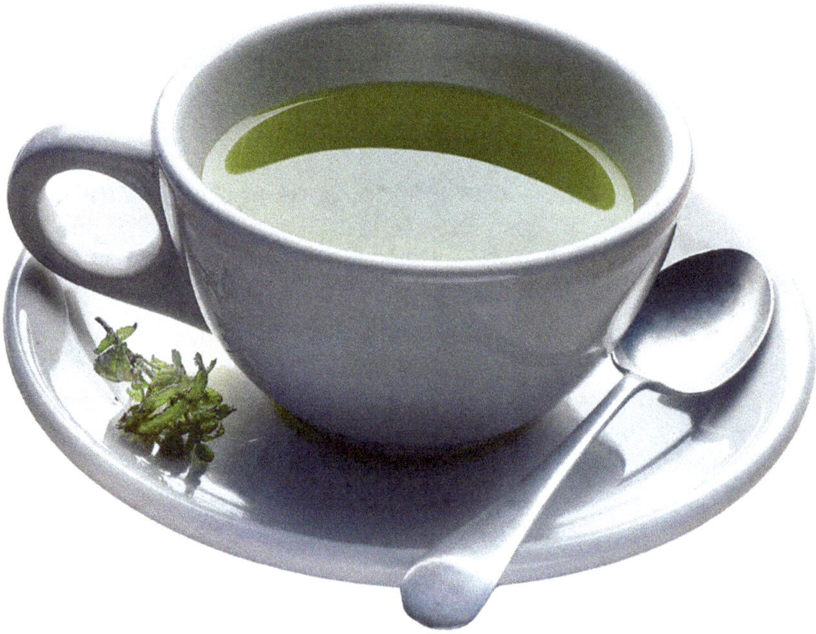

Green tea comes from unoxidized leaves of the Camellia sinensis bush. It is one of the least processed types of tea, containing the most antioxidants and beneficial polyphenols. Some research suggests green tea may positively affect weight loss, liver disorders, type 2 diabetes, Alzheimer's disease, and more.

Green Tea for Treating Lupus

Green tea is rich in antioxidants, polyphenols, and catechins, which may help reduce inflammation and improve immune function in lupus patients. However, while green tea can support overall health, it should be consumed in moderation as it may interact with certain lupus medications.

Health Benefits of Green Tea for Lupus

✓ Anti-Inflammatory Properties – Green tea contains EGCG (Epigallocatechin gallate), which helps reduce inflammation and prevent flare-ups.

✓ Boosts Immune System – It strengthens immune function, helping the body fight infections common in lupus patients.

✓ Supports Heart Health – People with lupus are at higher risk of heart disease, and green tea helps improve cardiovascular function.

✓ Protects Against Oxidative Stress – The antioxidants in green tea help protect cells from damage caused by free radicals.

How to Make Green Tea for Lupus

Ingredients:

- 1 teaspoon green tea leaves (or 1 tea bag)
- 1 cup hot water (not boiling, around 175°F or 80°C)
- Honey or lemon (optional)

Instructions:

1. Steep the green tea leaves (or bag) in hot water for 2-3 minutes.
2. Strain and add honey or lemon for taste (optional).
3. Drink 1-2 cups daily, preferably in the morning or afternoon.

Coconut milk (Parasite killer)

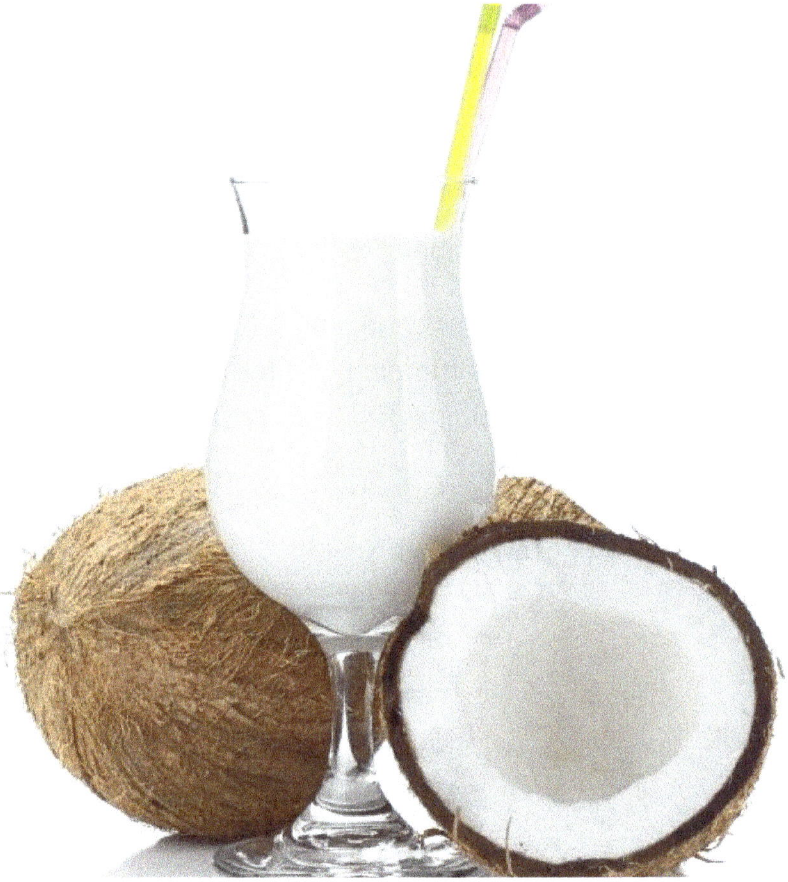

Yes, coconut milk—especially when paired with other parts of the coconut like the oil or flesh—can help support gut health and may assist in fighting parasites naturally.

How Coconut Milk May Help with Gut Parasites

- Contains Lauric Acid
- Coconut milk is rich in lauric acid, which the body converts into monolaurin, a compound known for its antimicrobial and antiparasitic properties.

- Monolaurin may help break down the outer membranes of certain parasites, bacteria, and fungi.

- Supports a Healthy Gut Microbiome
- Coconut milk can help maintain a healthy balance of gut flora, which is important for keeping parasites and bad bacteria in check.

- Soothing to the Digestive Tract
- Its anti-inflammatory properties can help calm the gut and reduce irritation that sometimes allows parasites to thrive.

How to Use Coconut Milk for Parasite Support:

- Drink 1 cup of pure coconut milk daily on an empty stomach for 5–7 days for stronger effect.
- Combine with 1 tbsp of coconut oil, which is even higher in lauric acid.
- Add grated raw garlic or papaya seeds (also known for antiparasitic effects) to smoothies with coconut milk for a powerful natural cleanse.

Coconut milk is generally safe, but overconsumption may cause digestive upset in some people due to its fat content.

Pavana (Croton)

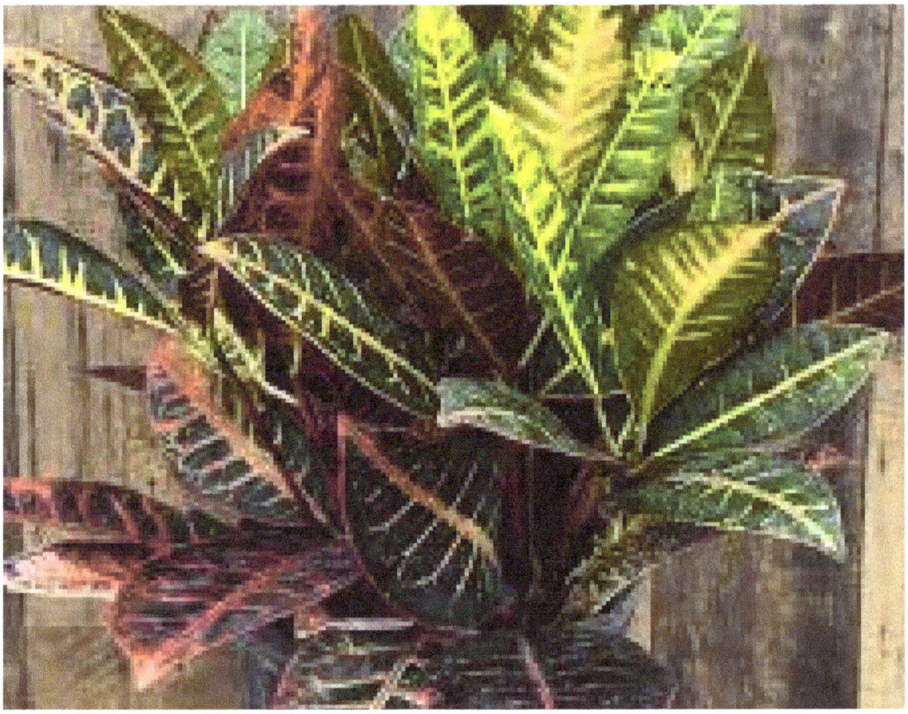

Pavana (Croton tiglium)—also known as Jamaican Croton, Purging Croton, or simply Croton—is a powerful herb traditionally used in folk medicine, particularly in Ayurveda and Caribbean herbal practices.

Health Benefits of Pavana (Croton tiglium)

Powerful Laxative (Purgative)

- Traditionally used to relieve severe constipation by stimulating intense bowel movements.
- Considered one of the strongest natural purgatives.
- Detoxification
- Helps cleanse the digestive tract by flushing out toxins.
- Sometimes used in detox regimes, but only in minute, diluted doses.
- Skin Conditions
- Used externally (not ingested) to treat skin infections, boils, and itchiness.

- The oil is sometimes applied to affected areas in extremely diluted form.

Worm and Parasite Expulsion

- Its purgative effects help remove intestinal worms and parasites naturally.
- Traditional Use in Cancer Treatment (Folk Remedies)
- In some traditional systems, it's been used in combination with other herbs for tumor reduction or anti-cancer protocols, though this is not supported by modern clinical research.

How to make Pavana leaf tea:

- Dried or fresh leaf
- add 2-3 leaves to 2 cups of water
- boil and simmer for few minutes
- (Optional) sweeten with sugar or honey

Lantana Camara

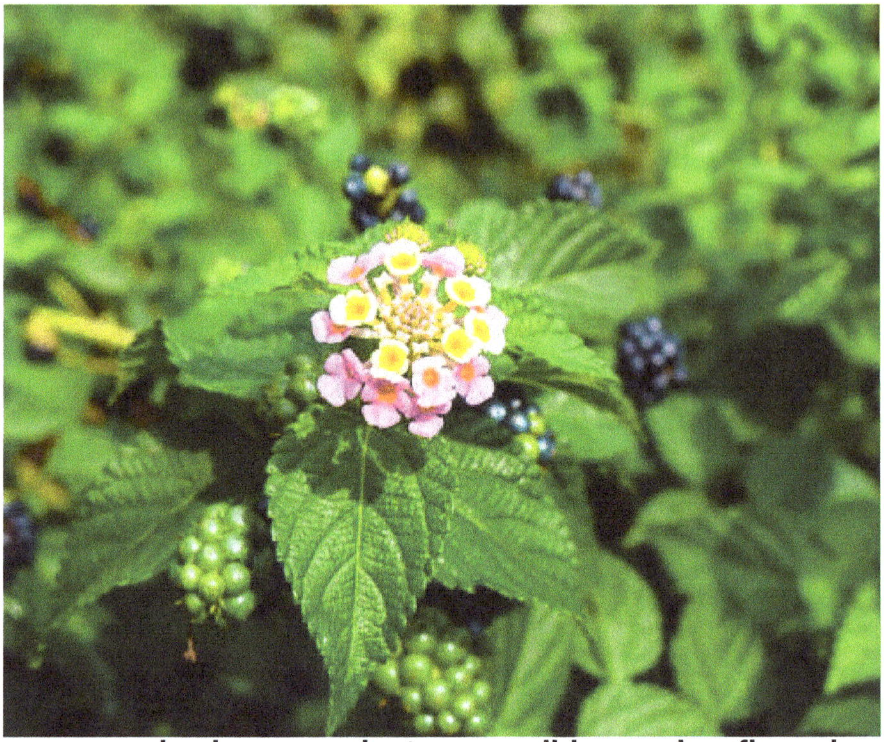

Lantana camara, also known as lantana or wild sage, is a flowering plant commonly found in tropical and subtropical regions.

is a flowering plant used traditionally in some cultures for its medicinal properties.

Health Benefits of Lantana Camara (Traditional Uses):

- **Anti-inflammatory properties:** In traditional medicine, Lantana camara has been used as an anti-inflammatory agent. It may help reduce swelling and inflammation when applied topically in the form of poultices or used in teas.

- **Antioxidant**: Lantana leaves and flowers have been shown to have antioxidant properties, which may help protect the body from oxidative stress and free radicals.

- **Antibacterial properties:** Some studies suggest that Lantana camara has antimicrobial properties and may help fight bacterial infections when used externally or in topical treatments.

- **Wound healing**: Traditionally, Lantana camara has been applied to wounds and ulcers. It is believed that the plant helps to speed up healing and reduce infection.

- **Digestive health**: Some people use Lantana leaves in herbal remedies for digestive issues like indigestion, bloating, or constipation.

. Respiratory Relief

- Some cultures use lantana leaves as an herbal steam to relieve cold symptoms, cough, or nasal congestion.

Antimicrobial Properties

- Extracts from the leaves have shown activity against various bacteria and fungi, making it useful in traditional medicine for wound cleaning or minor skin infections

How to Make Lantana Camara Tea (Traditional Method)

Ingredients:

- 2–3 fresh or dried lantana camara leaves (only the green leaves – avoid berries or woody stems)
- 1–2 cups of water
- (Optional) Honey or lemon for taste

Instructions:

1. Wash the leaves thoroughly to remove any dirt or contaminants.
2. Boil 1–2 cups of water in a small pot.
3. Add the washed lantana leaves.
4. Reduce heat and simmer for 5–7 minutes.
5. Turn off the heat and let it steep for another 5 minutes.
6. Strain the tea into a cup.
7. Add a bit of honey or lemon if desired, to improve the taste.

Red amaranth

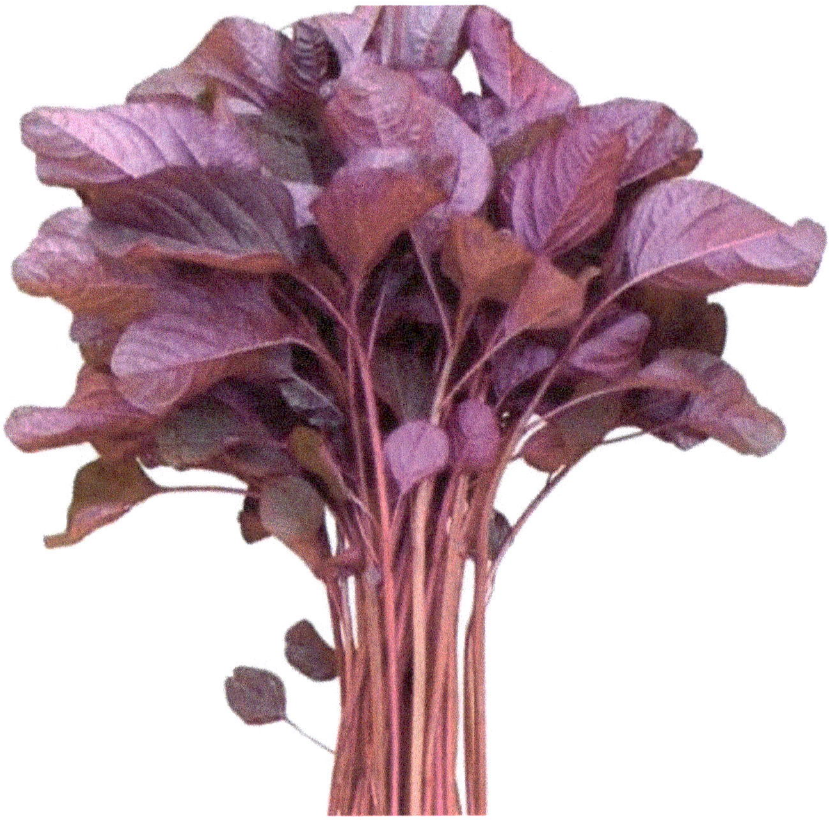

Amaranth leaves are a storehouse of essential nutrients. They are loaded with vitamins A, C, K, and folate, vital for supporting a robust immune system, promoting healthy vision, and aiding in cell growth and repair. Consuming amaranth leaves may benefit heart health.

The nutrients in amaranth can offer significant health benefits as part of a healthy diet. It's a source of vitamin C, which is vital to your body's healing because it helps process iron, form blood vessels, repair muscle tissue, and maintain collagen.

Here are some other health benefits of amaranth:

Naturally gluten-free

Amaranth is a good option for people with Celiac disease, a condition in which an immune system reaction to wheat gluten can damage the small intestine.

High in protein

Amaranth is one of the richest plant forms of protein available. The protein is easily absorbed by the body and contains all amino acids — even lysine, which is often missing from cereal grains. Studies show that in the plant kingdom, amaranth proteins are among the most similar to animal proteins.

Antioxidant-rich

Amaranth is rich in antioxidants, including gallic acid and vanillic acid. Antioxidants help fight free radicals, which are damaging byproducts of your body's normal cell activity, helping reduce everything from signs of aging to heart disease.

Eases inflammation

Some allergic reactions lead to uncomfortable inflammation through the production of immunoglobulin E. Early studies show that amaranth can slow down the body's production of immunoglobulin E.

Amaranth Leaves Benefits

Although amaranth is best known for its seeds, the leaves are edible, too.
The leaves are a source of several vital nutrients, including:

- Carotenoids
- Protein
- Dietary fiber
- Amino acids such as methionine and lysine
- Magnesium
- Calcium
- Potassium
- Copper
- Phosphorous
- Zinc
- Iron
- Manganese
- Vitamin C
- Beta-carotene

Amaranth leaves have many of the nutritional benefits of other greens, such as spinach or kale, and can be used the same way.
The antioxidants in amaranth leaves can help protect you against several conditions, including:

- Heart disease
- Cancer
- Arthritis
- Emphysema
- Cataracts
- Blocked arteries

Amaranth is a highly nutritious plant used as both a grain and leafy green. It's rich in protein, fiber, iron, magnesium, and antioxidants, and it's naturally gluten-free. You can use both the seeds and the leaves in your diet, depending on the health benefits you're looking for.

How to Use Amaranth Seeds (Grain)

- 1. Cook as a Whole Grain (like quinoa or rice)
- Ingredients:
- 1 cup amaranth
- 2.5–3 cups water or broth
- Pinch of salt

Instructions:

1. Rinse the amaranth seeds under cold water.
2. Bring water or broth to a boil.
3. Add amaranth and reduce heat to a simmer.
4. Cover and cook for 20–25 minutes, until water is absorbed and grains are soft.
5. Fluff with a fork and serve.

Great for porridge, grain bowls, soups, or as a side dish.

Make Amaranth Porridge

- Use 3 cups water or plant milk to 1 cup amaranth.
- Add cinnamon, vanilla, or fruit for flavor.
- Simmer for 25–30 minutes until thick and creamy.

Pop Amaranth (like popcorn)

- Heat a dry pan until hot.
- Add 1 tablespoon of dry amaranth seeds at a time.
- Cover and shake the pan until the seeds pop.
- Use as a crunchy topping on yogurt, salads, or snacks.

White pine

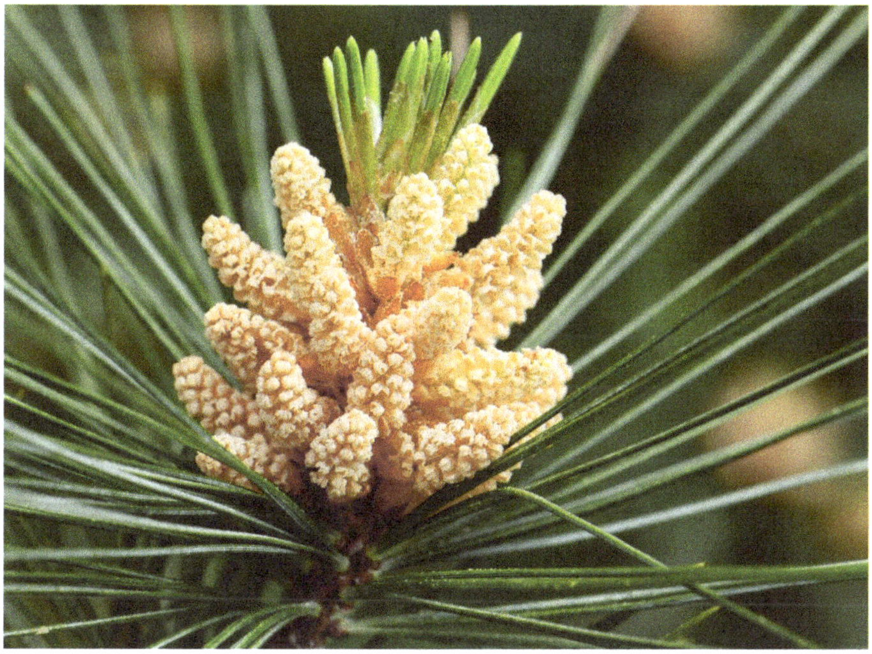

It's no wonder why white pine (Pinus strobus) is considered the majestic tree. Its majestic height makes it the largest pine tree in the US. This big and mighty tree packs an oversized punch of nutrients that can help u feel and look healthy. Since colonial times, both the colonists and British learned their lesson well about white pine and value it for its medicinal properties.

Historically, white pine lumber was employed by Americans and British for building ships. Except that it was the Americans who first realized that the inner bark of white pine could actually be consumed. However, the animals are always way ahead of their time and had known the nutritional value of white pine even before the advent of Americans.

For generations, white pine has served as a natural remedy for cough, chest congestion, bronchitis, laryngitis, and other upper respiratory tract infections. It is packed with impressive polyphenols that can help repair the damaged skin, tackles the wrinkles, and steps up the game of collagen and skin elasticity to give you younger-looking skin.

White Pine (Pinus strobus), also known as Eastern White Pine, has been used traditionally for its various medicinal benefits.
Here's a summary of its health benefits and ways to use it:

Respiratory Support

- Acts as an expectorant, helping to clear mucus from the lungs.
- Used in herbal teas or steam inhalation for colds, coughs, bronchitis, and sinus congestion.

Anti-inflammatory Properties

- Contains anti-inflammatory compounds that may help reduce swelling and pain, especially for sore throats and inflamed tissues.

Rich in Vitamin C

- The needles are a good source of Vitamin C, supporting immune health and combating fatigue or scurvy.

Antioxidant and Antimicrobial

- Pine contains antioxidants and may help fight off infections and support healing.

Urinary Tract Support

- Acts as a mild diuretic, promoting healthy urination and flushing of the kidneys and bladder.

How to Use White Pine

White Pine Needle Tea

Ingredients: A handful of fresh or dried white pine needles (avoid brown or old needles).

Steps:

- Chop the needles to release the oils.
- Boil water, then remove from heat.
- Add needles and steep for 10–15 minutes.
- Strain and drink. Add honey or lemon if desired.

Steam Inhalation

- Boil pine needles in water.
- Place your face over the pot (carefully) and cover your head with a towel.
- Inhale deeply for 5–10 minutes to clear nasal and chest congestion.

Salve or Poultice (External Use)

- Made from infused white pine in oil, useful for chest rubs or healing minor wounds.

White Pine and Erectile Dysfunction: What You Should Know

1. Improved Circulation

- White pine has vasodilatory (blood vessel-widening) properties due to its antioxidant content.
- Better blood flow is essential for erectile function.
- Its vitamin C content also supports blood vessel health and nitric oxide production.

2. Anti-Stress and Respiratory Support

- Stress, anxiety, and respiratory issues can affect sexual performance.
- Drinking white pine tea may offer calming effects and help reduce stress, which can indirectly support libido and performance.

3. General Immune and Hormonal Support

- Healthy testosterone levels and immune function are necessary for consistent sexual health.
- White pine's antioxidants may protect against inflammation that can negatively affect hormone balance.

Patchouli

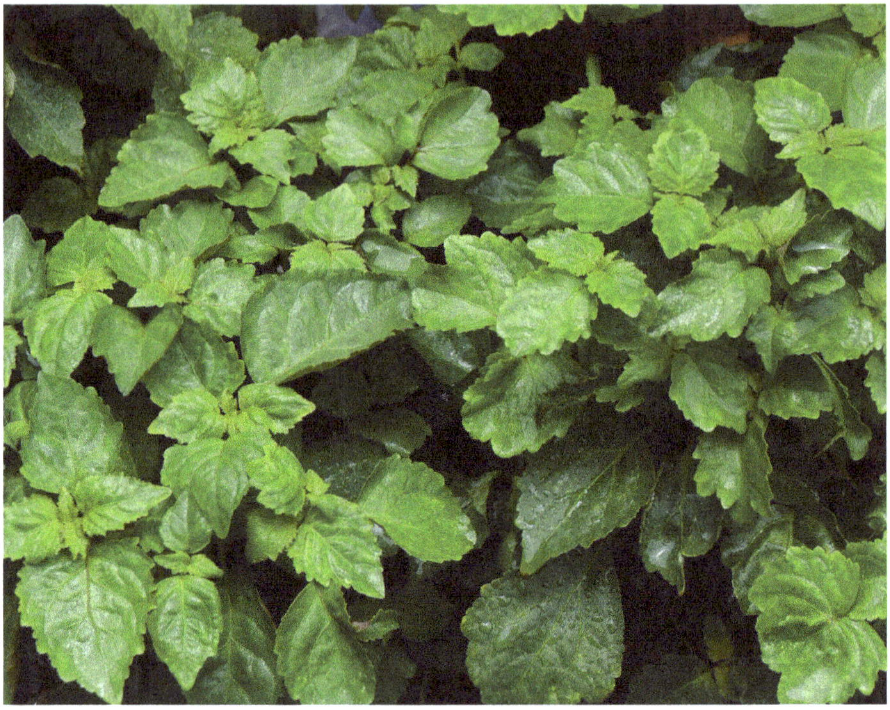

Patchouli (Pogostemon cablin) is best known for its deep, earthy fragrance, but it also offers a variety of health benefits — especially when used as an essential oil or herbal infusion. Here's a breakdown of its top medicinal properties:

Patchouli Health Benefits

1. **Mood Booster & Antidepressant**

- Patchouli oil has calming and grounding effects.
- It may help reduce stress, anxiety, and depression by promoting relaxation.
- Often used in aromatherapy for emotional balance.

2. **Anti-Inflammatory**

- Can reduce inflammation in conditions like arthritis or muscle pain.
- May help with swelling or irritation when diluted and applied topically.

3. **Antibacterial & Antifungal**

- Effective against bacteria like Staphylococcus aureus.
- Can treat fungal infections such as athlete's foot or dandruff.

4. **Skin Health & Anti-Aging**

- Promotes healing of wounds, scars, eczema, and acne.
- Stimulates new cell growth and reduces the appearance of wrinkles.

5. **Aphrodisiac**

- Traditionally believed to enhance libido and sexual desire.
- Used in sensual massage oils or in romantic settings.

6. **Insect Repellent**

- Natural alternative to chemical repellents for mosquitoes and bugs.
- Can be diffused or added to sprays for skin or home use.

7. **Immune System Support**

- May stimulate immune function thanks to its antimicrobial properties.

8. **Digestive Aid** (Traditionally)

- In traditional Chinese medicine, patchouli is used to help with indigestion, nausea, and diarrhea.

Patchouli Tea for Digestion Problems

Digestive Benefits:

- Relieves Nausea – Especially helpful if caused by motion sickness or stomach bugs.
- Eases Bloating & Gas – Acts as a mild carminative.
- Supports Digestion – Stimulates digestive enzymes and bile flow.
- Helps with Diarrhea & Vomiting – Used traditionally to stabilize digestion during stomach infections or food poisoning.
- Calms the Stomach – Gentle on the digestive tract and may reduce inflammation.

How to Make Patchouli Tea for Digestion

Ingredients:

- 1–2 teaspoons dried patchouli leaves (or a small fresh sprig)
- 1 cup of hot water
- Optional: a slice of ginger or a dash of honey for extra digestive support

Instructions:

1. Bring water to a boil and remove from heat.
2. Add patchouli leaves and steep for 5–10 minutes.
3. Strain and sip slowly.
4. Drink once or twice a day as needed for digestive relief.

Trumpet leaf (Kidney repair)

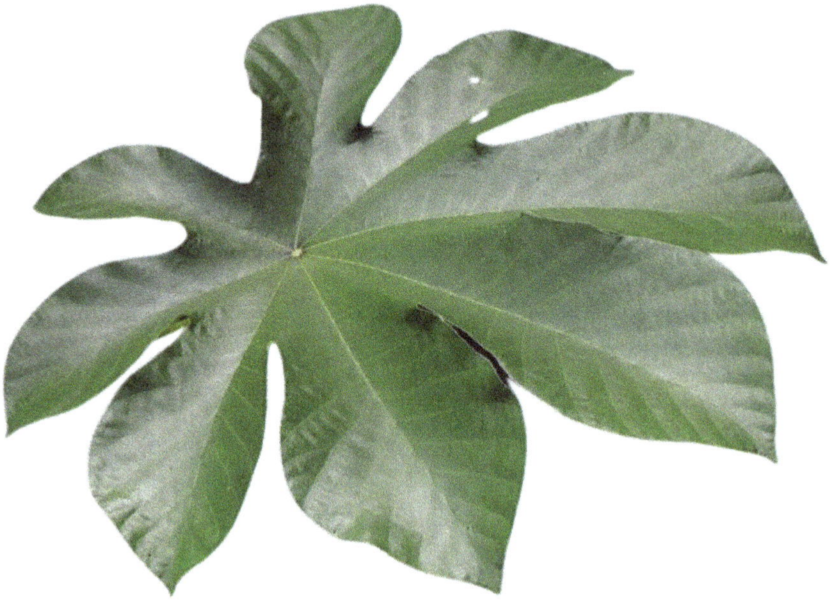

In traditional Jamaican and other cultures, trumpet tree leaves (Cecropia peltata) are used for various medicinal purposes, including treating respiratory issues, managing diabetes, and supporting kidney function, with potential benefits as an antioxidant and anti-inflammatory agent.

Traditional Uses and Potential Benefits:

Respiratory Support:

- Used to alleviate cough, cold, and asthma symptoms.
- May help soothe throat irritation and promote easier breathing.
- Diabetes Management:
- Traditional use suggests they can help regulate blood sugar levels.
- Some compounds in the leaves, like anthranilic acid, may lower blood glucose levels.
- Kidney Function:
- May promote urination and support kidney function.

Anti-inflammatory and Antioxidant Properties:

- Possess anti-inflammatory properties, potentially reducing inflammation and swelling. Rich in antioxidants, which help combat oxidative stress.

Other Traditional Uses:

- May be used to treat liver ailments and dropsy.
- Used to treat hypertension, heart conditions, and nervous diseases.
- Used to treat back pain.
- Used to treat skin infections.
- Used to treat dysentery.
- Used to treat bronchitis, obesity, bacterial infection, and respiratory disorders.
- Used to treat Parkinson's disease.
- Used to treat cold and flu.
- Used for Parkinson disease

To make trumpet leaf tea, boil fresh or dried trumpet leaves (Cecropia peltata) in water for several minutes, strain, and then drink the tea warm. You can use about one teaspoon of dried leaves per cup of hot water.

Here's a more detailed guide:

- Gather your leaves: You can use either fresh or dried trumpet leaves.
- Boil water: Bring fresh water to a full boil.
- Add the leaves: Place about one teaspoon of dried leaves (or a handful of fresh leaves) into a pot or cup of boiling water.
- Steep the tea: Allow the leaves to steep in the hot water for several minutes, allowing the healing compounds to infuse into the liquid.
- Strain the tea: Remove the leaves and strain the tea to remove any remaining debris.
- Serve and enjoy: Drink the tea warm, often several times a day, to address specific health concerns.

Fagara zanthoxyloides (Sickle cell)

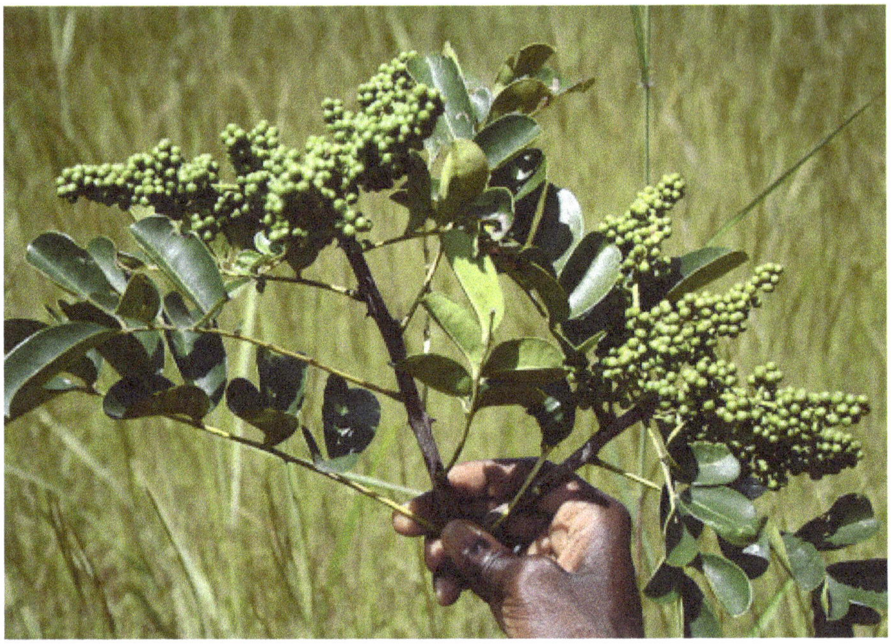

Fagara zanthoxyloides (also known as Zanthoxylum zanthoxyloides) has been traditionally used in some regions to treat sickle cell anemia, and research suggests that compounds from its root bark, like divanilloylquinic acids, exhibit antisickling properties.

Traditional Use:

Zanthoxylum zanthoxyloides is a plant species in the Rutaceae family, and its different parts (fruits, stem bark, leaves, and roots) have been used in traditional medicine for various ailments, including sickle cell anemia, fever, malaria, tumors, and pain management.

Antisickling Properties:

Studies have investigated the antisickling effects of compounds isolated from the root bark of F. zanthoxyloides.

Divanilloylquinic Acids:

Researchers have identified three isomeric divanilloylquinic acids (burkinabin A, B, and C) in the root bark of F. zanthoxyloides.

Other Traditional Uses:

Besides sickle cell anemia, Zanthoxylum zanthoxyloides has been used traditionally to treat or manage conditions like trypanosomiasis, malaria, microbial infections, tuberculosis, and enteritis.

Fagara (Zanthoxylum zanthoxyloides) is traditionally used in African herbal medicine, especially for managing sickle cell disease. It's known for its anti-inflammatory, antioxidant, and analgesic properties.

How to Consume Fagara Safely

- 1. Decoction (Root Tea)
- Ingredients:
- 1–2 tablespoons of dried Fagara root (shredded or chopped)
- 2 cups of water

Instructions:

1. Add the roots to water and bring to a boil.
2. Let it simmer for 20–30 minutes.
3. Strain and drink 1/2 cup once or twice daily.

Powdered Form

- Grind dried root into powder.
- Mix 1/2 teaspoon into warm water, honey, or smoothies.
- Take once daily.

Dong Quai

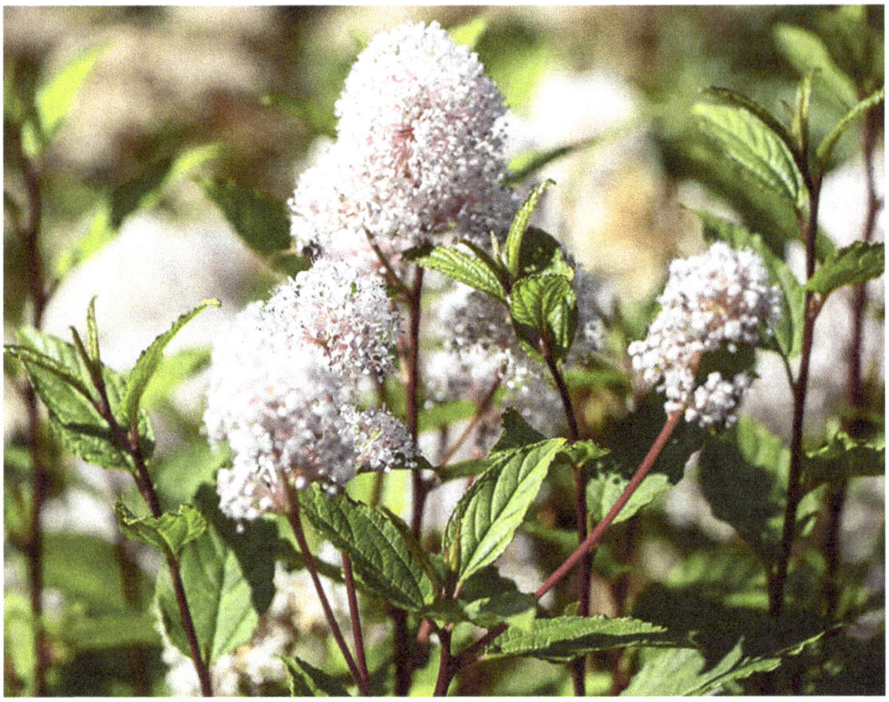

Dong quai, also known as Angelica sinensis, is a traditional Chinese herb used for various purposes, primarily related to women's health, including menstrual cramps, menopausal symptoms, and promoting blood circulation.

Here's a more detailed look at its uses and potential benefits:

Traditional Uses and Potential Benefits:

Menstrual Issues:

- **Dysmenorrhea** (painful menstruation): Dong quai is often used to alleviate menstrual cramps and pain.
- **Irregular Menstrual Cycles**: It may help regulate menstrual cycles and address issues like amenorrhea (absence of menstruation) or scanty periods.
- **Premenstrual Syndrome** (PMS): Dong quai is sometimes used to manage symptoms of PMS, such as breast swelling, bloating, and mood swings.

Menopause:

- **Menopausal Symptoms:** It is traditionally used to help alleviate symptoms associated with menopause, including hot flashes and night sweats.
- **Hormonal Balance**: Dong quai is known for its hormone-balancing properties, which can be beneficial during menopause.

Hormonal Balance:

It's often referred to as "female ginseng" and is believed to have hormone-balancing properties.

Other Potential Uses:

- In traditional Chinese medicine, dong quai is also used for conditions like:
- Anemia: It's believed to help build blood and enhance hormonal functioning.
- Joint Pain: It may have anti-inflammatory effects that can help alleviate joint pain.
- High Blood Pressure: Some suggest it can help manage hypertension.
- Allergies: It's used in the prevention and treatment of allergic attacks.
- Skin Conditions: Some believe it can help with skin dryness and promote a healthier complexion.
- Cancer: Some studies suggest that dong quai may have potential anti-cancer properties, but more research is needed.

Drug Interactions:

Dong quai may interact with certain medications, including blood thinners, so it's important to talk to your doctor before taking it, especially if you have any medical conditions or are taking other medications.

Pregnancy and Breastfeeding:

Dong quai is generally not recommended during pregnancy or breastfeeding due to potential risks.

How to Make Dong Quai Tea

Ingredients:

- 1–2 teaspoons of dried Dong Quai root (Angelica sinensis)
- 2 cups of water
- Optional: honey, ginger, or lemon for flavor

Instructions:

1. Rinse the root (if whole or sliced) to remove dust or impurities.
2. Add Dong Quai to 2 cups of water in a saucepan.
3. Bring to a boil, then reduce heat and let it simmer for 20–30 minutes.
4. Strain the tea into a mug.
5. Add honey or lemon if desired.
6. Drink 1 cup once daily, ideally during the second half of your menstrual cycle (days 14–28), or as recommended by a herbalist.

Red Clover

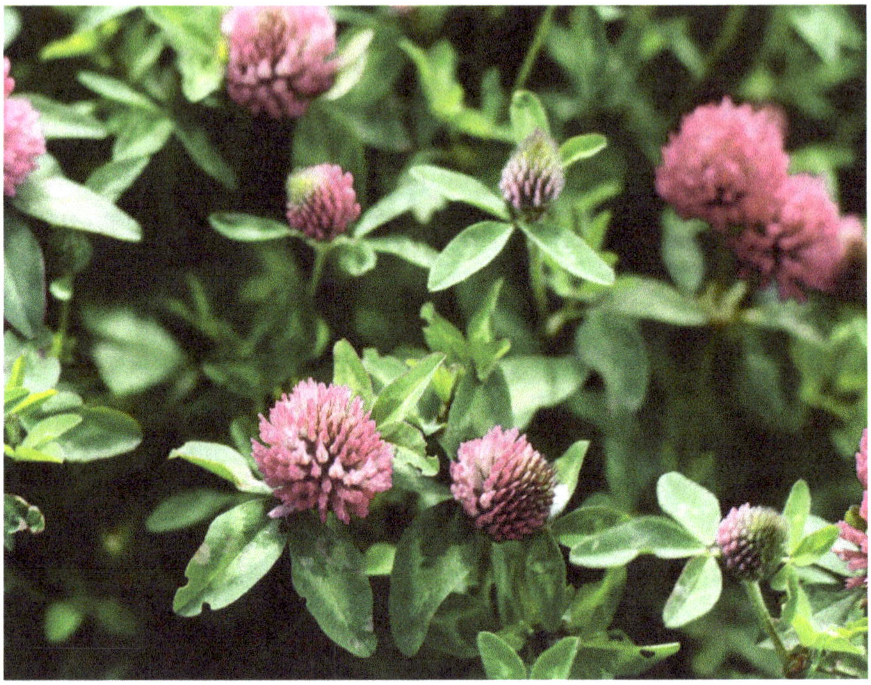

Red clover has also become a popular ingredient in shampoos and hair treatments to support hair health. In fact, research done by Obstetrics and Gynecology International reveals that red clover extract may even increase hair growth for those experiencing hair loss due to alopecia.

Red Clover Scalp Rinse / Tea

Ingredients:

- 2 tablespoons dried red clover flowers
- 2 cups boiling water

Instructions:

1. Steep red clover in boiling water for 15–20 minutes.
2. Let it cool completely.
3. After shampooing, pour the tea over your scalp and massage gently.
4. Leave it in or rinse out after 10–15 minutes.
5. Use 2–3 times per week.

Benefits: Stimulates hair follicles, reduces inflammation, and promotes scalp circulation.

Red Clover-Infused Oil

Ingredients:

- ½ cup dried red clover flowers
- 1 cup carrier oil (like coconut or jojoba)

Instructions:

1. Place red clover and oil in a glass jar.
2. Let it infuse in a warm place for 1–2 weeks or heat gently for a quicker infusion.
3. Strain and store in a dark bottle.
4. Massage into the scalp 2–3 times weekly.

Benefits: Nourishes hair roots and strengthens follicles.

Internal Use (for Hormonal Support)

Red Clover Tea

- Steep 1 teaspoon of dried red clover in 1 cup hot water for 10–15 minutes.
- Drink once daily.

Benefits: Supports hormonal balance (especially in estrogen-related hair loss in women), detoxifies blood, and promotes hair growth from within.

Precautions:

Avoid during pregnancy or breastfeeding.

Not recommended for people with hormone-sensitive conditions (e.g., breast cancer, fibroids).

Always consult your doctor if taking blood thinners or hormone therapies.

Marshmallow root

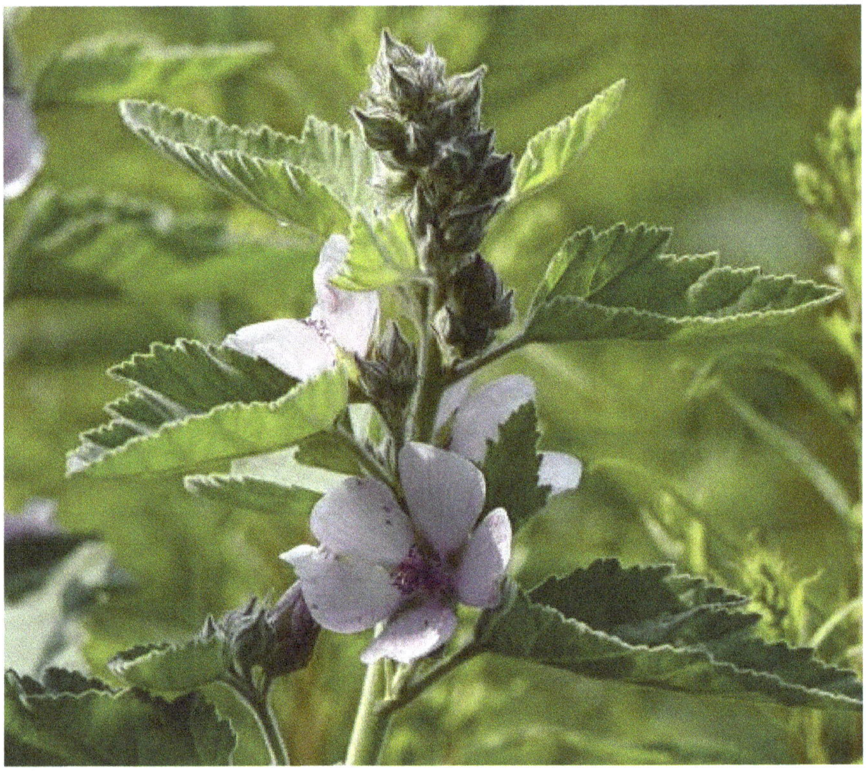

Marshmallow root, known as Althaea officinalis, offers potential health benefits including soothing irritated skin, aiding digestion, and supporting respiratory health, thanks to its mucilaginous and anti-inflammatory properties.

Here's a more detailed look at the potential health benefits of marshmallow root

Respiratory Health:

- Sore Throat and Cough Relief: Marshmallow root's mucilage coats the throat, soothing irritation and reducing the urge to cough.

- Dry Cough: The mucilage helps lubricate the throat, which can help with dry coughs.

- Respiratory Issues: Marshmallow root may help with conditions like bronchitis and laryngitis.

Digestive Health:

Gut Soothing:

- The mucilage coats the lining of the digestive tract, protecting it from irritation and inflammation.

Digestive Issues:

- It may help with conditions like gastritis, ulcers, and inflammatory bowel disease.

- Promotes Tissue Regeneration:

- Marshmallow root can promote tissue regeneration, protecting the lining of the digestive tract.

Skin Health:

- Soothing Irritation: Marshmallow root can help soothe irritated skin, wounds, and burns.

- Hydration and Repair: It contains skin-protecting polysaccharides that help hydrate and repair the skin.

- Inflammatory Skin Conditions: Marshmallow root may help with conditions like eczema and psoriasis.

Anti-inflammatory:

- It has anti-inflammatory properties that can help reduce inflammation in the body.

Kidney Health:

- Marshmallow root may help reduce inflammation in the kidneys and urinary tract.

Urinary Tract Infections:

- It can help soothe the lining of the urinary tract and increase urine flow, potentially helping with UTIs.

Hair Health:

- Marshmallow root can hydrate and soften hair, making it easier to detangle and reduce frizz.

Here's how to make soothing and healing marshmallow root tea — an herbal remedy commonly used for sore throat, cough, digestive issues, and urinary tract health. Marshmallow root is rich in mucilage, a gel-like substance that coats and soothes irritated tissues.

How to Make Marshmallow Root Tea

Ingredients:

- 1 tablespoon dried marshmallow root
- 1 cup cold or room temperature water
- Optional: honey or cinnamon for taste

Cold Infusion Method (Best for sore throat & gut health)
This method preserves the mucilage content.

- Place 1 tablespoon of dried marshmallow root into a glass jar or cup.
- Pour 1 cup of cold water over it.
- Cover and let it steep for at least 4–8 hours, or overnight.
- Strain the root out.
- Sweeten with a little honey if desired. Drink 1–2 times daily.

Poke root & Castor Oil

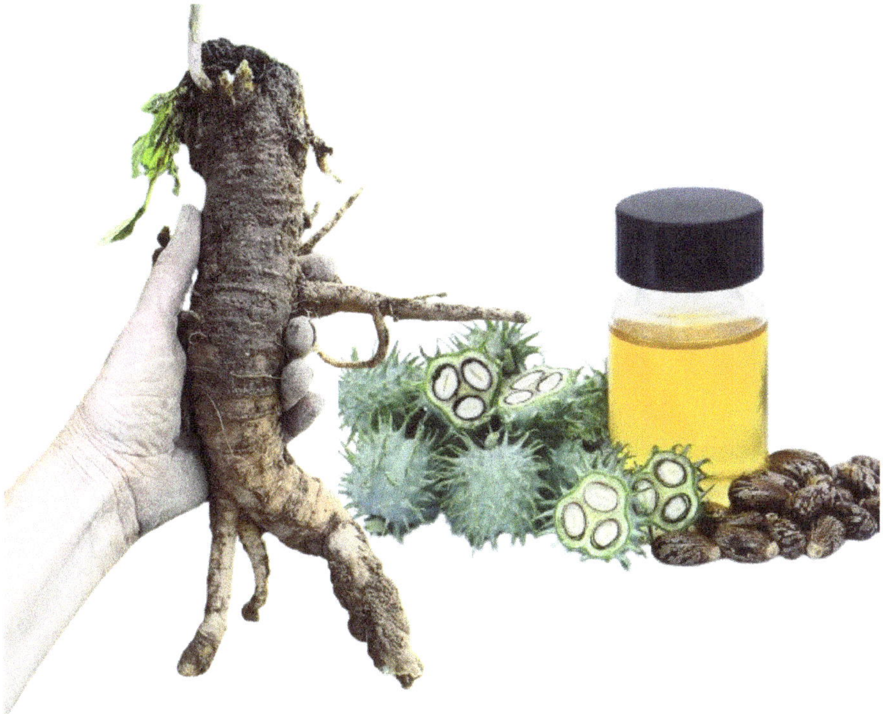

Poke Root (Phytolacca americana) and Castor Oil (Ricinus communis) are powerful natural remedies traditionally used for detoxification, lymphatic drainage, inflammation, and skin conditions. When used together—especially topically—they may provide deep healing benefits. However, both are potent and must be used with care.

Relieves Pain & Swelling

- Applied to joints, abdomen, or swollen areas for relief from arthritis, menstrual cramps, or digestive issues.
- Heals Skin Conditions
- Used for dry skin, scars, cysts, and infections.

Poke Root + Castor Oil Pack (For Lymphatic Swelling or Cysts)

Ingredients:

- 1–2 drops of poke root tincture or infused oil
- 1 tablespoon castor oil
- A piece of flannel or cotton cloth

Instructions:

1. Mix poke root (just a drop or two) with castor oil.
2. Soak the cloth in the mixture.
3. Apply to the affected area (like swollen lymph nodes, cysts, or joints).
4. Cover with plastic wrap and a heating pad.
5. Leave on for 20–45 minutes.
6. Use once daily for several days.

Turkey berry

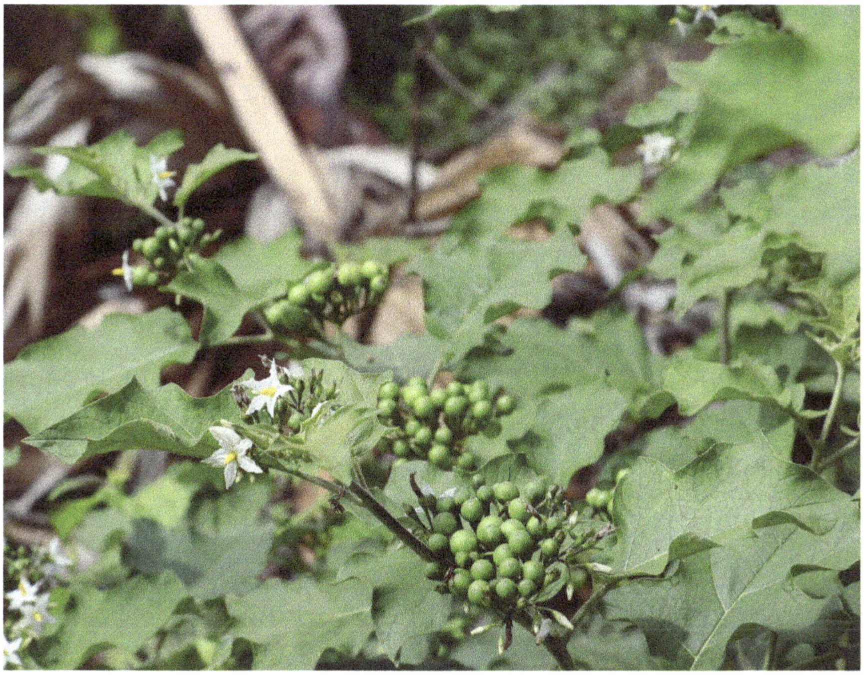

Turkey berry, also known as Solanum torvum, offers potential health benefits, including aiding digestion, potentially treating anemia due to its iron content, and possessing antioxidant and anti-inflammatory properties.

Here's a more detailed look at the potential benefits of turkey berry

Improves Digestion:

- Turkey berry is believed to aid digestion and may help with indigestion, stomachaches, and diarrhea.

Neutralizes Stomach Acid:

- The antioxidants in turkey berry, like phenols and chlorogenins, may help neutralize stomach acids, potentially beneficial for conditions like gastritis or ulcers.

Fiber Content:

- The high fiber content in turkey berry can facilitate smooth digestion, promote weight loss, and maintain a normal appetite.

Other Potential Benefits:

Anemia Treatment:

- Turkey berry is a good source of plant-based iron, which can be helpful in treating or preventing iron deficiency anemia, although absorption may vary.

Blood Sugar Control:

- Turkey berry may help regulate blood sugar levels, making it potentially beneficial for individuals with diabetes.

Cardiovascular Health:

- Turkey berry may contribute to cardiovascular health by helping regulate blood pressure and reducing inflammation.

Kidney Health:

- Turkey berry may help flush out uric acid, which could be beneficial for kidney health and potentially prevent or minimize symptoms of gout.

The ample antioxidant content in turkey berry, of phenols and chlorogenins, help to neutralize stomach acids in situations of intestinal gastritis or pancreatic ulcers. Moreover, the massive fibre content facilitates smooth digestion of food, accelerates weight loss and maintains normal appetite.

To make turkey berry tea, simply steep 1-2 teaspoons of dried turkey berry leaves (Solanum torvum) in 8 oz of hot water for 5-10 minutes, then strain and enjoy.

Here's a more detailed breakdown:

- Gather your ingredients: You'll need dried turkey berry leaves (Solanum torvum) and hot water.
- Prepare the water: Heat water to a boil, then let it cool slightly to a temperature that's hot but not scalding.
- Add the leaves: Place 1-2 teaspoons of dried turkey berry leaves in a cup or teapot.
- Steep the tea: Pour the hot water over the leaves and let it steep for 5-10 minutes.
- Strain and serve: Strain the tea to remove the leaves and enjoy.
- Optional: You can add honey or other sweeteners to taste.

Carrot leaves

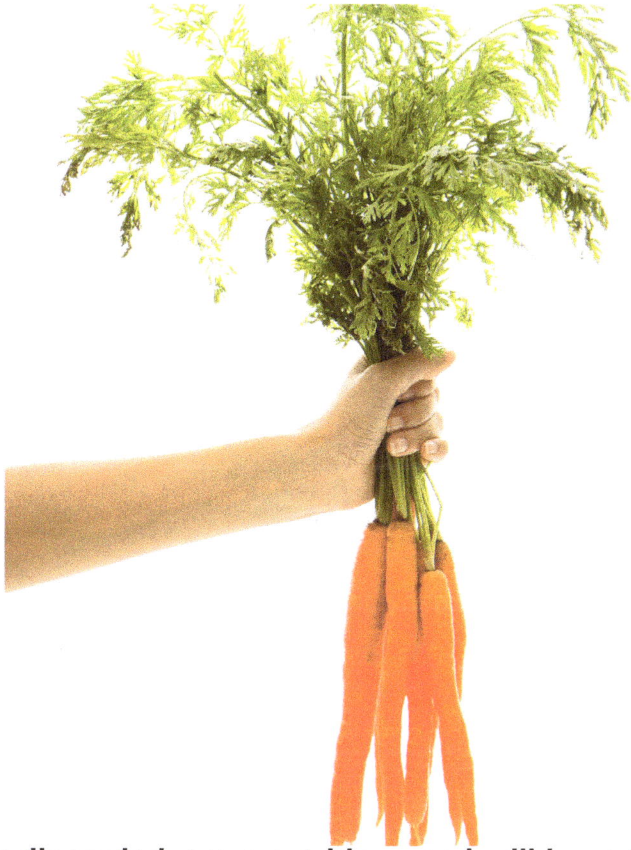

Carrot leaves, often discarded, are a nutritious and edible part of the carrot plant, offering benefits like being a good source of vitamins (A, C, K), minerals (potassium, calcium), fiber, and antioxidants, potentially supporting digestive health, immune function, and overall well-being.

Here's a more detailed look at the benefits of carrot leaves

Vitamins:

- Vitamin C: Carrot tops contain significantly more vitamin C than the root, about six times more.
- Vitamin A: They are a good source of beta-carotene, which the body converts into vitamin A, essential for vision and immune function.
- Vitamin K: Important for bone health and blood clotting.
- Minerals:
- Potassium: Important for maintaining healthy blood pressure.
- Calcium: Essential for strong bones and teeth.
- Magnesium: Plays a role in muscle function and nerve transmission.

Potential Health Benefits:

- **Improved Digestive Health:** The fiber content in carrot leaves can contribute to a healthy digestive system by preventing constipation and supporting regular bowel movements.

- **Enhanced Immune Function:** The vitamins and minerals in carrot leaves can contribute to a healthy immune system, helping the body defend against infections and illnesses.

- **Bone Health**: The presence of vitamin K in carrot leaves is beneficial for bone health, as vitamin K is essential for proper blood clotting and plays a role in bone metabolism.

- **Reduced Risk of Chronic Diseases**: A diet rich in nutrients, including those found in carrot leaves, has been associated with a reduced risk of chronic diseases.

- **Blood Sugar Regulation**: The fiber content in carrot leaves can help regulate blood sugar levels.

- **Detoxification:** Chlorophyll in carrot leaves may support the detoxification process.

How to Incorporate Carrot Leaves into Your Diet:

- Wash Thoroughly: Before using, wash the carrot leaves thoroughly under running water to remove any dirt or debris.

- Chop Finely: Chop the leaves finely and add them to salads, soups, stews, or other dishes.

- Use as Seasoning: Use them as a fresh, slightly bitter seasoning for various dishes.

- Add to Smoothies: Blend them into green smoothies for an extra nutrient boost.

- Infuse Tea or Water: Infuse carrot leaves in tea or water for a flavorful and healthy beverage.

Jamaican Sarsparilla root

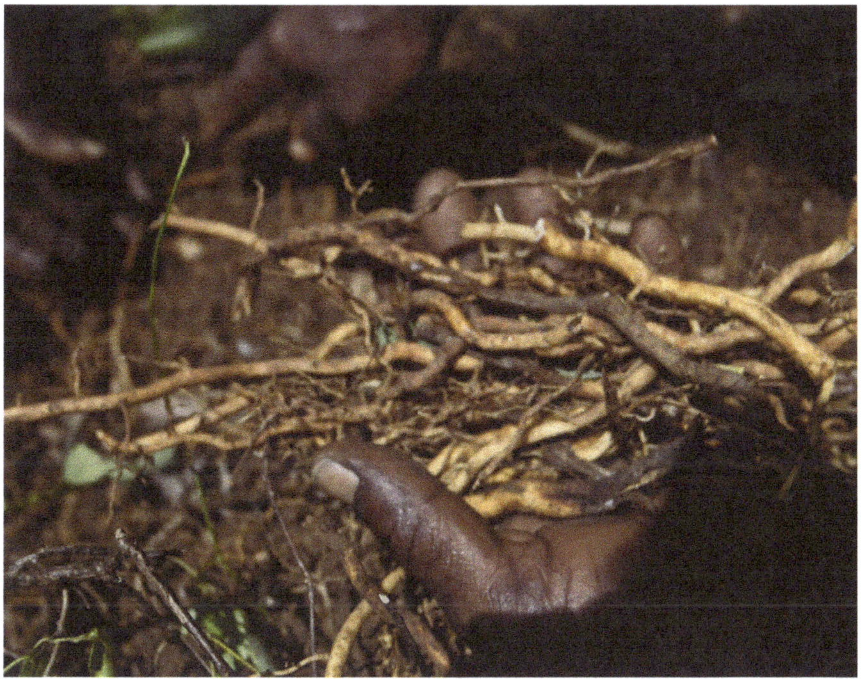

Sarsparilla is a tropical plant used throughout history to treat conditions like arthritis, psoriasis, and syphilis.

Sarsaparilla is a tropical plant from the genus Smilax. The climbing, woody vine grows deep in the canopy of the rainforest. It's native to South America, Jamaica, the Caribbean, Mexico, Honduras, and the West Indies.

For centuries, indigenous people around the world used the root of the sarsaparilla plant for treating joint problems like arthritis, and for healing skin problems like psoriasis, eczema, and dermatitis. The root was also thought to cure Hansen's disease (leprosy) due to its "blood-purifying" properties.
Sarsaparilla was later introduced into European medicine and eventually registered as an herb in the United States Pharmacopoeia to treat syphilis.

The benefits

Sarsaparilla contains a wealth of plant chemicals thought to have a beneficial effect on the human body. Chemicals known as saponins might help reduce joint pain and skin itching and also kill bacteria. Other chemicals may help reduce inflammation and protect the liver from damage.

1. **Psoriasis**

The benefits of sarsaparilla root for treating psoriasis were documented decades ago. One study found that sarsaparilla dramatically improved skin lesions in people with psoriasis. The researchers hypothesized that one of sarsaparilla's main steroids, called sarsaponin, is able to bind to endotoxins responsible for the lesions in psoriasis patients and remove them from the body.

2. **Arthritis**

Sarsaparilla is a potent anti-inflammatory. This factor makes it also a useful treatment for inflammatory conditions like rheumatoid arthritis and other causes of joint pain and the swelling caused by gout.

3. **Syphilis**

Sarsaparilla has shown activity against harmful bacteria and other microorganisms that have invaded the body. Though it may not work as well as modern day antibiotics and antifungals, it has been used for centuries to treat major illnesses like Hansen's disease (leprosy) and syphilis. Syphilis is a sexually transmitted disease caused by a bacterium. Hansen's disease (leprosy) is another devastating infection caused by bacteria.

The antimicrobial activity of sarsaparilla has been documented in recent studies. One paper looked at the activity of over 60 different phenolic compounds isolated from sarsaparilla. Researchers tested these compounds against six types of bacteria and one fungus. The study found 18 compounds that demonstrated antimicrobial effects against the bacteria and one against the fungus.

4. **Protecting the liver**

Sarsaparilla has also shown protective effects on the liver. Research conducted in rats with liver damage found that compounds rich in flavonoids from sarsaparilla was able to reverse damage to the liver and help it function at its best.

5. **Improving the bioavailability of other supplements**

Sarsaparilla is used in herbal mixes to act as a "synergist." In other words, it's thought that the saponins found in sarsaparilla increase the bioavailability and absorption of other herbs.

How to Make Sarsaparilla Tea: Easy Recipe

Ingredients

- 1/4-1 tsp shredded sarsaparilla root
- 8 ounces hot water
- honey/sugar (optional)

Instructions

1. Chop and shred the pieces of the root as finely as possible.
2. Bring a saucepan of water to boil.

Coral vine

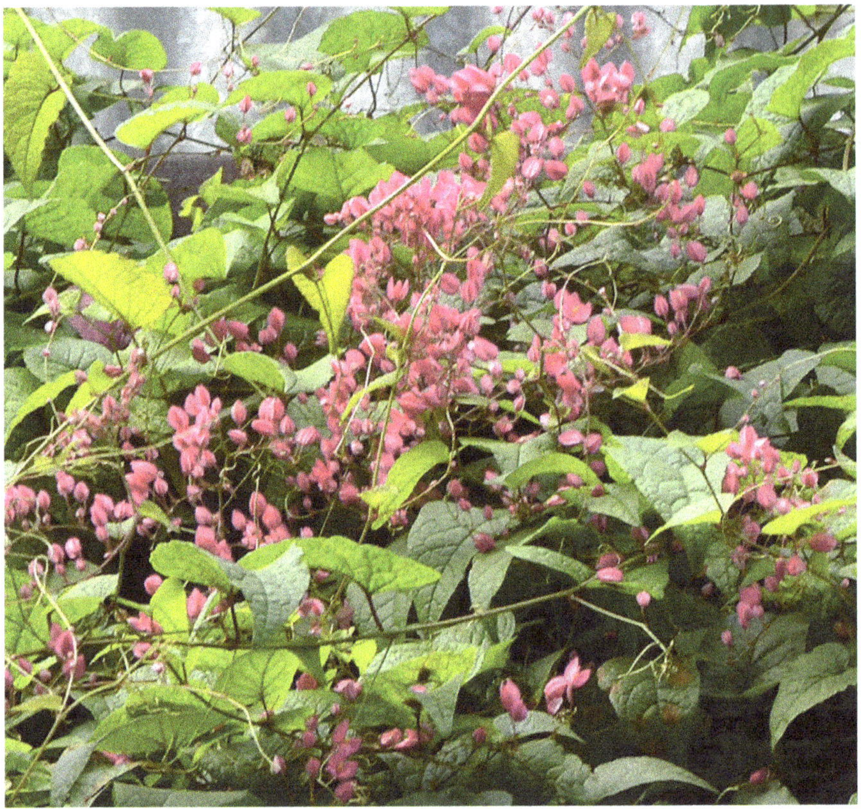

This herb possesses several therapeutic properties. A tea made from the coral vine's aerial parts is used to cure common cold and also provide relief from pain. The aerial parts of coral vine are collected and dried and later used to prepare a hot tea for curing flu and sore throat.

Coral vine is used for multiple purposes, including therapeutic and food. This herb possesses several therapeutic properties.
A tea made from the coral vine's aerial parts is used to cure common cold and also provide relief from pain. The aerial parts of coral vine are collected and dried and later used to prepare a hot tea for curing flu and sore throat.

Findings of several studies have shown that the aerial parts of coral vine can be effective in treating cold, diabetes, reduce swellings, healing wounds and also for providing relief from pain. In addition, the tea can also be used in the form of a heart tonic.
An extract of the leaves and flowers of this plant has the ability to slow down the process of lipid peroxidation. It has been established that this plant possesses anti-inflammatory, antioxidant and analgesic properties.

Coral Vine Tea (Antigonon leptopus) & Its Health Benefits

Coral Vine, also known as Mexican creeper, chain-of-love, or Antigonon leptopus, is a beautiful climbing plant with pink or white flowers. In traditional herbal medicine, especially in the Caribbean, Philippines, and parts of Asia, coral vine tea is valued for its gentle yet effective health-supporting properties.

How to Make Coral Vine Tea

Ingredients:

- 1–2 teaspoons of dried coral vine leaves or flowers (or a mix)
- 1–2 cups of hot water
- Optional: honey, lemon, or ginger for taste

Instructions:

1. Boil water and pour over the dried coral vine parts.
2. Let steep for 10–15 minutes.
3. Strain and enjoy warm or cool.
4. Drink once or twice daily.

Health Benefits of Coral Vine Tea

1. Anti-inflammatory

- Helps reduce joint pain, muscle aches, and other inflammation-related symptoms.
- Traditionally used to ease arthritis and similar conditions.

2. Antioxidant-Rich

- Contains compounds that fight free radicals, supporting skin health, immune strength, and anti-aging.

3. Fever Reduction

- Often used in folk medicine as a natural remedy for fevers, especially in children.

4. Respiratory Support

- May help soothe symptoms of coughs, sore throats, or chest congestion.

5. Wound Healing Support (External Use)

Ginger and Garlic tea (Herpes)

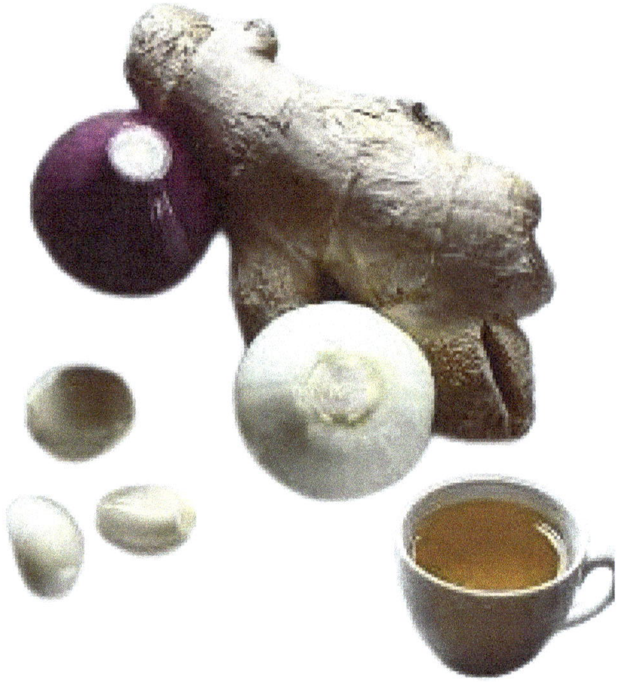

Yes, absolutely! You can boil onion and ginger together to make a powerful herbal tea that supports your immune system and may help manage herpes symptoms naturally. While it won't cure the virus, this tea can help your body fight outbreaks, reduce inflammation, and ease discomfort.

Onion & Ginger Immune Tea (Herpes Support Blend)

Ingredients:

- 1 small red or yellow onion (sliced or chopped)
- 1–2 inches of fresh ginger root (sliced or grated)
- 2–3 cups of water
- Optional: juice of ½ lemon, raw honey (for taste and added benefit)

Instructions:

1. Add sliced onion and ginger to a pot with 2–3 cups of water.
2. Bring to a boil, then simmer for 15–20 minutes.
3. Strain the tea into a cup.
4. Add lemon juice and honey if desired.
5. Drink 1 cup, once or twice daily during outbreaks or as daily immune support.

Benefits:

Onion: Antiviral, high in quercetin (which may inhibit HSV), boosts immunity.

Ginger: Reduces inflammation, improves circulation, relieves pain and discomfort.

Lemon & Honey (optional): Add vitamin C and extra soothing properties.

Tips & Precautions:

Drink warm for best results.

If you have acid reflux, drink after meals to avoid irritation.

Not a replacement for medication if you're on antiviral treatment—this is a supportive remedy.

🌿 Special Thank You

I extend my deepest gratitude to every single person who has supported Eternal Life in Plants — whether by purchasing a copy, sharing it with a friend, or simply taking the time to explore its pages.

Your belief in this work means more than words can express. This book was written with love, intention, and reverence for the healing power of nature, and it is truly an honor to share it with you.

To those who connected with the message, felt inspired by the knowledge, or found even a moment of peace or clarity within these pages — thank you. You are the reason this book exists.

May the wisdom of plants continue to bring life, light, and healing to your journey.

With sincere appreciation,

Donovan Broderick

Author

www.ingramcontent.com/pod-product-compliance
Lightning Source LLC
LaVergne TN
LVHW080039210926
848481LV00011B/3231